Health Manpower and Productivity

Health Manpower and Productivity

The Literature and Required Future Research

Edited by
John Rafferty

Lexington Books
D.C. Heath and Company
Lexington, Massachusetts
Toronto   London

Grateful acknowledgment is made to the American Medical Association for permission to reprint various tables and quotations that have been copyrighted by the American Medical Association in 1966, 1967, 1968, 1969, 1970, 1971 and 1972.

Library of Congress Cataloging in Publication Data

Rafferty, John, 1935-
   Health manpower and productivity.

   1. Medical personnel—United States. I. Title. [DNLM: 1. Health manpower—U.S. W76 R137h]
RA410.7.R33   331.1'26   74-13403
ISBN 0-669-95521-3

Published simultaneously in Canada.

Printed in the United States of America.

International Standard Book Number: 0-669-95521-3

Library of Congress Catalog Card Number: 74-13403

To Lise

Contents

List of Figures   ix

List of Tables   xi

Foreword
   Herbert E. Klarman   xiii

Introduction
   John Rafferty   xxi

Part I   *Issues in Health Manpower Productivity*

Chapter 1   **Manpower Substitution in Ambulatory Care**
                      Uwe E. Reinhardt and *Kenneth R. Smith*   3

Chapter 2   **Productivity and Economies of Scale in
                      Medical Practice**
                      Richard M. Scheffler   39

Chapter 3   **Effects of Incentives on Physician
                      Performance**
                      Frank A. Sloan   53

Chapter 4   **Patient Participation and Productivity
                      in the Medical Care Sector**
                      Fredrick L. Golladay   85

Chapter 5   **A Review of Productivity in Dentistry**
                      Paul J. Feldstein   107

Chapter 6   **Occupational Licensure and Health Care
                      Productivity: The Issues and the
                      Literature**
                      H.E. Frech   119

viii

Part II   *A General Overview*

Chapter 7   **Research on Health Manpower Productivity:**
                     A General Overview
                     Jack Hadley   143

                     Index   205

                     About the Contributors   227

List of Figures

1-1   Transforming Two Inputs into One Output   6

1-2   Physician Input vs. Aide Input   7

1-3   Line Slope between Two Processes
       Representing Rate of Input
       Substitution   8

1-4   Total Product Curves for Aide Utilization
       by Physicians   19

1-5   Physician Usage of Pediatric Nurse
       Practitioners   27

List of Tables

1-1   Staffing Patterns for Managing 120
          Particular Patient Visits per Week   20

2-1   Median Net Incomes, Solo Practitioners,
          and Numbers of Partnerships, 1962-1966   47

3-1   Group Management   64

3-2   Groups by Method of Income Distribution   65

3-3   Method of Income Distribution: Ratio to
          Equal Income Sharers to Varying Income
          Sharers by Size and Type of Group   65

3-4   Weeks Worked, Visits, and Expenses per
          Visit   68

3-5   Hours of Work by Type of Practice and
          Specialty   72

3-6   Mean Incomes by Practice Type   74

3-7   Practice Mode Preferences or Residents
          When the Decision Is Made   76

3-8   Factors Influencing Practice Mode Choice
          by Type of Practice Selected   77

3-9   Major Deterrents to Careers in Private
          Practice, Hospital Practice, and
          Academic Medicine as Viewed by
          Physicians in Residency Programs   78

5-1   Average Annual Patient Visits per Dentist
          by Number of Auxiliary Personnel
          Employed   109

6-1   Medical Schools, Students, and Graduates:
          1905-1960   124

6-2	Black Physicians and Physicians of All Races: 1890-1969	125
6-3	Number of Predominantly Jewish City College of New York Graduates Admitted to Medical School: 1929-1943	126
7-1	Rates of Change of Death Rates and Hospital Use, 1948-1968	154
7-2	Production Functions for Private Practitioners	158
7-3	Performance and Delegation of Office, Technical, Laboratory, and Clerical Tasks as Reported by Pediatric Practitioners, U.S.A.	160
7-4	Office Patient Care Tasks According to Present Performance and Opinion about Their Delegation	161
7-5	Extent of Present Delegation to Allied Health Workers and Extent to Which Internists Believe Delegation Should Be Made	162
7-6	Bailey's Findings	173
7-7	Pediatricians	175
7-8	Practice Size and Productivity Relationships	176
7-9	Hospital Staff Physicians	176
7-10	Weeks Worked, Visits, and Expenses for Visits	177
7-11	Hours Worked and Visits per Week	180
7-12	Variations in Patient-Visit Rates by Location	185

Foreword

This collection of papers, originally commissioned by the Bureau of Health Services Research of the Health Resources Administration (of the U.S. Department of Health, Education, and Welfare), partakes of the time-honored tradition of the survey paper or monograph. Such a survey, whether in economics or in the health services, represents an effort to review the state of knowledge concerning a given problem or subject area. By summarizing what investigators have reported and by comparing their findings, the reader is able to distill the factual foundations for policy recommendations and to establish baselines and points of departure for further research. Thus, a successful review paper is rooted in both relevant theory and empirical research; it summarizes what is known and indicates what is not known; and it formulates questions to be asked and approaches toward answering them.

A useful review paper yields still another benefit. Owing to its wide scope, it sometimes draws on two or more disciplines and usually draws on several subspecialties within a discipline. Of necessity, professional jargon is translated into the common parlance of the English language, thereby enabling the intelligent layman or interested policy-maker to read in depth and with understanding about issues and technical controversies that lie outside his normal compass.

The volume's title, *Health Manpower and Productivity*, is self-explanatory. The focus is on the productivity of health manpower, on ways to improve the ratio of output to manpower input in the health services industry. Efficiency in the use of manpower is important, regardless of the level of demand for health services relative to supply, now and in the future. The reason is the very rationale for the pursuit of economics: in a world in which people have more wants than the totality of resources can meet, any savings that accrue from more efficient production can be put to worthwhile uses. There is a second reason, perhaps peculiar to the health field: if it is true, as many students of the health services contend, that the supply of resources is a major determinant of the demand for health services, then studies of personnel requirements that are based on medical need (as determined by biological factors plus the capabilities of technology) or even on some set of autonomous forces of demand (wants, however derived, supported by purchasing power) have lost practical meaning. It has become desirable, perhaps necessary, to shift the emphasis of study, as well as of policy, in the health field to the supply side of the equation.

It is simple to show that, owing to the persistent power of compound interest, an increase in the productivity of manpower by 2(3) percent a year is the same as an increase in numbers by 22(34) percent in 10 years and by 49(81) percent in 20 years. Accordingly, there can be no doubt that a survey of the literature on health manpower is potentially useful. What serves to make such a survey useful in fact is the accumulation of a sufficient volume of pertinent literature, adequate in technical proficiency, which awaits review, analysis, and evaluation. It was the judgment of John Rafferty, the editor of this volume, that the time was ripe for such an undertaking. For this writer, Rafferty's judgment has been vindicated by the collection of studies at hand.

Description

Of the seven chapters, one—Feldstein's—deals with productivity in dental care. It is a summary of a particular dimension of the economics of dentistry—those gains in productivity that are attainable through labor intensive approaches. Feldstein discusses the gains ensuing from the introduction of additional auxiliary personnel into dental practices in this country and of better-trained, expanded-function auxiliaries in New Zealand. He explicitly excludes here other sources of productivity gain, such as improved technology, which are dealt with in his full scale monograph.[1]

It is noteworthy that Feldstein acknowledges that the measurement of output in dental care is less complex than the measurement of output in medical care. This point has received increasing recognition since its elucidation in Jeffrey H. Weiss's work on productivity in dentistry and in nursing.[2]

The remaining chapters deal with productivity in the provision of medical care to ambulatory patients (in-patient services are not considered).

Three chapters are lengthy—Reinhardt and Smith on production functions and activity analysis; Sloan on incentives to the individual physician as the size of the medical practice varies; and Hadley's overview, which may serve both as a summary of the other chapters and as a synthesis of certain technical problems, such as the quality of care and capital substitution.

Among the shorter chapters, Scheffler's is technical, and draws attention to the valid distinction between productivity comparisons in different settings, organizational or other, and economies of scale, which pertain to variation in physical productivity or cost in the long run, as the size of firm changes. Clearly this distinction is important where a comparison is attempted between single- and multi-specialty medical practices. As Scheffler points out, its empirical findings on the latter would bear on the HMO (Health Maintenance Organization).

The other two shorter chapters are essentially exploratory essays, dealing with potential sources of productivity gains that have not yet been treated in the empirical health economics literature. Golladay, writing on patient participation, draws on such diverse sources as medical sociology, health education, epidemiology, and medical care. Frech, in the chapter on licensure, draws on economic theory, the economics of industrial structure, history of the professions, public health, and the law of regulation.

Summary of Findings

The following seem to be the major points developed in the six chapters on the productivity of health manpower in the delivery of medical care to ambulatory patients.

1. The two major sources of increase in physician productivity after World War II are (1) the shift away from house calls toward office visits, hospital care, and consultation by telephone; and (2) advances in biomedical knowledge and technology, especially in the widespread application of the antibiotic drugs.

2. A steady substitution of auxiliary health manpower for physicians has continued to take place. Indeed, it is now technically feasible for physicians to make appreciably greater use of auxiliary manpower than they actually do, thereby enhancing their own and total health manpower productivity. This conclusion derives support from a number of studies that employ different approaches and different sets of data. Estimated continuous production functions indicate that the average solo practitioner in medicine could profitably employ twice as many auxiliary health workers as he does—four instead of two, increasing the number of patient visits per physician per week by 25 percent. An activity analysis of how primary medical care practice should be organized finds that the productivity of individual physicians could be increased by 75 percent through the use of physicians' assistants.

In an attempt to present a more coherent picture of the literature on health manpower productivity, Reinhardt and Smith offer a bold synthesis of the findings for pediatric services, in which they consider possibilities of substitution among all types of health manpower, those that are primarily supportive of the physician and those that may replace him in part. They also show the relationship between the older production function and the newer, discrete activity analysis. For the future they envisage a larger role for activity analysis, which will require the collection of large masses of data in the clinical setting.

3. Technical feasibility, however, is not tantamount to economic feasibility. To begin with, there is the obvious matter of relative wages among the several health manpower categories that can serve as substitutes for one another. Technical feasibility represents an increase in physically measured output per unit of input. There is economic feasibility when the value of the increase in output exceeds the cost of the proposed substitution.

4. Laws and regulations, particularly licensure, may be obstacles to the substitution of health manpower. As Hadley points out, the magnitude of such an effect is not known. Frech offers a measure of excess earnings in medicine, which is presumptive of restriction of entry into the occupation. Such measures have a time-honored history, beginning with the pioneer study of professional incomes by Friedman and Kuznets.[3] It is fair to add, however, that such measures continue to be fraught with controversy, both as to size and as to the causal factors they reflect.[4] The description of economic discrimination is graphic but dated.

Frech discusses certification and institutional licensure as less restrictive alternatives to personal licensure. He also mentions the possibility of licensure examinations that are open to all, without any educational prerequisite.

5. Larger firms may afford greater opportunities for manpower substitution,
owing to the presence of indivisibilities among factors of production.

6. In larger medical practices with cost sharing and income sharing, however, the
individual physician stands to gain less and less from gains in efficiency. As the size
of firm increases, incentives toward efficiency facing the individual, autonomous
physician steadily diminish. Such disincentives may be overcome by moving toward centralized decision-making and by moving away from equal income shares.
Sloan introduces some data, but they do not bear directly on the hypotheses being
tested.

Moreover, the available data either confound the factors of practice size and of
method of reimbursement or have nothing to say about how the individual physician is paid. Hadley's conclusion is accurate, that the empirical evidence on the
effect of alternative reimbursement mechanisms on physician productivity is practically nonexistent. Rather, what is believed to be known derives from economic
theory and reasoning from anecdotal experience.

7. Capital substitution for manpower is certainly a technical possibility. According to Hadley, much of the work on capital in recent years has centered on the
computer and has been done by engineers and computer specialists. They tend not
to ask the types of questions asked by economists about benefits in relation to
costs or about cost-effectiveness. Often they seem to favor adoption of the best
prevailing practice.

It is fair to note that the cost-benefit literature on the health services does
contain examples of capital substitution other than the computer.[5] However, they
pertain mostly to the hospital, which has historically served as the locus for the
bulk of social capital invested in the health field. Opportunities for capital investment in facilities for ambulatory patients remain to be explored.

The notion of the best prevailing practice appears to have a dual meaning. On
the one hand, it is a standard of the quality of care. On the other hand, it is
employed as a guide to the types and range of services that ought to be made
available to a population. In Hadley's example of hemodialysis for persons with
end-stage kidney disease, the issue is not quality of care but a public policy decision
on how many and who will be eligible to receive such services.

8. As a logical extension of the concept of the physician extender, still another
source for increasing health manpower productivity is an increase in participation
by the patient or his family. Possible means of participation are: health maintenance; preventive medical services, as through periodic health examinations;
prompt seeking of care for diagnosis and treatment; compliance with the prescribed medical regimen; and reliance on the patient's and family's inputs, especially in chronic illness. This literature falls outside of economics, and hence is not
evaluated systematically by Golladay for possible contributions to empirical esti-

mates of productivity gains. It is unlikely that the existing literature can provide answers to specific questions from another discipline.

9. If productivity gains accrue, who will benefit? No answer can be ventured even on theoretical grounds without specific knowledge of the structure of the industry in a given time or place. If consumers organize and become large purchasers of medical care who face large medical practices, the situation becomes one of bilateral monopoly. In that case information is needed on the relative bargaining power of the parties, on public opinion, and on the knowledge available to each party concerning the other party's preferences.

Some Comments

All the chapters discuss one or more constraints on health manpower substitution, that is, the reasons that actual substitution falls short of the substitution that is said to be technically feasible. It may be that certain real constraints are underestimated.

Reinhardt and Smith touch upon the stochastic nature of the demand for a good deal of medical care, although they do not elaborate on it. Undoubtedly the extent of substitution and delegation is less when demand varies at random than when the production process is schedulable and routine. How much less is a question of fact.

Economists increasingly take account of the factor of time in explaining the demand for medical care. In the context of stochastic variation, time is of obvious importance: who will do the waiting, the provider or the patient?

Perhaps another constraint on substitution is the need for direct supervision by a physician. Although existing laws and practices may be too confining, the circumstances under which supervision may be waived are still to be spelled out. It may be useful to pursue further the implications of Reinhardt and Smith's distinction between physician supporters and physician substitutes.

In this context it is helpful to recall an unusual feature of the health services industry—consumer ignorance. It furnishes the basis for the relationship of agency, whereby the provider undertakes to act in the interests of the patient. Perhaps worthiness to participate in such a responsible relationship of trust is associated with long and arduous professional education and training. As Solow puts it, "Diplomas and degrees [may] function in part as a kind of signaling or screening device for certain traits and habits. . . ."[6]

Creative and original as Sloan's study is, its findings are naturally constrained by its assumptions. One assumption is that the input value of the physician's own time is a constant. What would be the implications of allowing the value of the physician's time to vary or change as his income increases? There is some reason to believe that the supply of labor by physicians bends backward after a certain level of income is attained.[7]

Reference was made earlier to the possible role of supply as a determinant of demand. If the proportions of health manpower are changed, what would be the possible effects on the level and patterns of health services utilization, apart from those associated with productivity? This question is obviously for the future.

Meanwhile, the chapters at hand display a healthy preoccupation with the measurement of output and a serious concern over the quality of care. A consensus emerges that in the context of productivity, measurement output is best viewed as an intermediate bundle of services, rather than as a change in health status. Quality of care is taken to be uniform, for lack of information to the contrary. The potential benefits of conducting joint research with clinicians, who are presumably expert in the quality area, are noted.

Obviously clinicians and other physicians can contribute to the understanding and measurement of the care of the art and science of medicine. But now it would be helpful to try and separate certain features of medical care that tend to fall under the rubric of quality. For example, privacy, promptness, and courtesy of service have value because they yield satisfaction to patients. However, they can be costed and priced separately from the core of quality. As the concept of quality is reduced, it will lend itself better to reliable and valid measurement.

Conclusions

This collection of papers is laudable in several respects:

1. It brings together the fragmented literature on health manpower productivity. Specific studies are analyzed and comparative findings are synthesized. Although the focus is on the physician, he is shown in relationship to other health workers.

2. The format of the volume has resulted in some duplication among the papers, especially between Hadley's and the others. An advantage of this duplication is that important points are made more than once and expressed in the differing languages of algebra, geometry, and English.

3. Some new data are presented and old data are reworked.

4. Many interesting questions are posed, some old and some new. A few old ones are put into a new and unexpected content.

5. Some hypotheses are accompanied by suggested approaches for empirical testing.

6. What is known is summarized and what is not known is made clear. The very strength of a survey volume is also its weakness: it can only report on what is found in the literature.

Notes

1. Paul J. Feldstein, *Financing Dental Care: An Economic Analysis* (Lexington, Mass.: Lexington Books, D.C. Heath and Company, 1973).

2. Jeffrey H. Weiss, "The Changing Structure of Health Manpower" (unpublished Ph.D. dissertation, Harvard University, 1966).

3. Milton Friedman and Simon Kuznets, *Income from Independent Professional Practice* (New York: National Bureau of Economic Research, 1945).

4. Herbert E. Klarman, "Approaches to Health Manpower Analysis, with Special Reference to Physicians" *The American Economist*, Vol. 17, No. 2 (Fall 1973), pp. 137-42.

5. Herbert E. Klarman, "Application of Cost-Benefit Analysis to Health Systems Technology," in *Technology and Health Care Systems in the 1980's*, edited by Morris F. Collen (Washington, D.C.: U.S. Government Printing Office, 1973), pp. 225-50.

6. Robert M. Solow, "Comment," in *The Measurement of Economic and Social Performance*, edited by Milton Moss (New York: National Bureau of Research, 1973), pp. 102-5; p. 103.

7. Martin S. Feldstein, "The Rising Price of Physicians' Services," *Review of Economics and Statistics*, Vol. 52, No. 2 (May 1970), pp. 121-33.

Introduction

The containment of rapidly increasing medical care costs has become a dominant policy objective, not just for the federal government, but for many state and local governments as well. A number of avenues for achieving this objective are under active consideration: the formal direct controls that had been introduced have now been abandoned, but a variety of reimbursement experiments are in progress, and other approaches of varying promise are presently being explored. Among these, there is strong hope that some moderation of rising medical care costs may result from efforts to increase manpower productivity in the health services sector. The degree to which there exists a real potential for such increases in productivity, however, remains a crucial and open question. It is that question which originally gave rise to this volume.

All of the contributions to this volume were initially commissioned in response to a specific need on the part of the federal government. During 1973 a broad, joint effort was expended by agencies of the Department of Health, Education, and Welfare to develop a Comprehensive Health Manpower Strategy, and one element in that effort dealt with the issue of manpower productivity. Responsibility for that topic fell to the National Center for Health Services Research and Development, the predecessor of the present National Center for Health Services Research. Part of that responsibility was met by a series of papers which provided background on the subject of manpower productivity. Although the original effort was to provide input for a Department report, it was apparent that the materials that were developed had the potential for becoming useful to a much broader audience. The present volume is the result.

The book has more than one purpose, and it is meant to address more than one audience. First, it provides an intensive critical review of past research, primarily in economics, dealing with health manpower productivity. This material is of interest particularly to economists, and should be especially useful to those economists who are new to the health field. In addition, however, the volume provides a relatively nontechnical analysis of the research results in this field, and this is aimed primarily at the noneconomist reader; it provides a useful synopsis of the information on health manpower productivity which economic research has been able to provide to date. Some economists, in addition, might find this nontechnical overview a useful and efficient introduction to the more technical aspects of the volume.

Finally, the volume places strong emphasis on needed future research. First, by reviewing past work, it attempts to provide the perspective that may lead to fruitful lines of future inquiry; it also presents much original thinking, and this, along with the perspective provided by literature review, leads to explicit research suggestions on each topic. It is hoped that this emphasis on needed future work will be useful in particular to the increasing number of new economists who are directing their attention to research in the health services sector, although it should also be of value to noneconomist researchers in allied fields.

The volume is developed in two parts. Part I consists of original technical papers on each of several specific areas which pertain to manpower productivity. Part II is a nontechnical overview of the entire field. From the perspective of some readers it might seem preferable to treat this overview as an introduction to the more technical individual papers; however, since the individual papers were commissioned first, with the overview written to draw heavily from them, there was some question of propriety. I have chosen to give the primary position to the original papers, with the overview as Part II of the volume, knowing that some readers will prefer to approach the book in the reverse sequence.

Few considerations in the health manpower field seem to offer as much promise for improvements in health services delivery as does substitution among manpower types. Concern for these possibilities has had its origins in the repeated projections of physician shortages in the United States; substitution of the services of nonphysician medical personnel for the services of physicians appears to be one of very few viable alternatives. More recently there has been talk of an impending physician surplus, but there is as yet little sign of agreement: estimated target dates at which a "surplus" in some sense may appear vary, and the possible effects of intervening variables on both supply and demand have not been consistently evaluated. Projections depend, among other things, on changes in specialty mix and on the extent of the increased demand for physicians' services that is expected to result from introduction of National Health Insurance. And, to whatever degree we do reach a surplus of physicians in an aggregate sense, no solution is in sight for distributional problems, especially shortages in central cities and rural areas. In addition, apart from these concerns with access, there is likely to be continued concern with rising medical care costs—and manpower substitution is one of the few modifications to our existing system that seems to hold much promise. Consequently, the volume begins with a treatment of this subject by two economists, Uwe Reinhardt and Kenneth Smith, whose work has been among the most prominent in this field. Their focus is upon technical feasibility of substitution between manpower types, and they review both the relevant production theory and the pertinent institutional settings. Past work is then reviewed, leading to a suggested approach for synthesizing various pieces of research. Suggested avenues for future research are then discussed.

One cornerstone of the present Administration's health policy has been the Health Maintenance Organization; development of HMOs has been effected via direct federal financial support, and is encouraged in the Administration's NHI proposal—the Comprehensive Health Insurance Plan. The main features of an HMO are *prepayment* and *group* rather than solo medical practice, and the latter of these two features is dealt with in Chapter 2, by Richard Scheffler. Again, the pertinent analytical framework is briefly reviewed and the literature on productivity of group practice and on economies of scale is examined; the author then identifies the central research problems and, as is the case in all subsequent chapters, he suggests the approaches that seem promising.

Elements of the financial side of group practice are then taken up in Chapter 3, by Frank Sloan. The author, who has done a substantial volume of research dealing with the behavior of physicians, here develops interesting models of physician decision-making. He deals, specifically, with implications of alternative arrangements for cost and revenue sharing in group practices, and he discusses both the implications of the models and the available institutional evidence. Then, in conjunction with the literature review, future research topics are presented.

While it is reasonable to focus primarily on physicians and paraprofessional substitutes for physicians in the context of questions dealing with health manpower productivity, the two subsequent chapters shift this focus to other pertinent issues. In Chapter 4, Fred Golladay addresses the subject of the patient's own input in the medical care process—the substitution of services by patients and their families for the services of professional providers. The author here surveys a field which has to date received only the most limited attention from the perspective of economics; drawing from a broad literature, the issues he discusses include the effects of patient participation on health status, activities aimed at prevention, problems of patient compliance, self-care, and effects of patient education. Chapter 5, by Paul Feldstein, then examines a second nonphysician topic, one which has also received only limited attention from economists, that of productivity in the field of dentistry. While supply limitations have not been a visible problem here, as they have for physicians, the importance of gaining further understanding of the dental sector has become more apparent in the context of National Health Insurance: there has been a growing possibility of inclusion of dental services in an NHI plan, and therefore there is the likelihood of a large increase in demand for these services. Chapter 5 reviews this topic, therefore, and suggests the more promising areas for research.

Chapter 6, by Ted Frech, is the final chapter of Part I. This deals with the very broad and pervasive issue of physician licensure, another topic which has received limited attention from economists. As the author points out, the effects of even modest changes in licensure terms or conditions might be expected to dominate the effects of other policy changes, and it is an area which continues to offer interesting analytical challenges for economists as well as for other investigators.

Part II, the general overview of the current state of knowledge pertaining to health manpower productivity, is written by Jack Hadley. This chapter offers a critical survey of a large volume of literature, drawing freely from the first six chapters as well as from numerous additional sources. It offers the reader—economist and noneconomist alike—a concise view of present knowledge on this topic, and the most promising areas for future research. As mentioned above, the inclusion and placement of this chapter gives the book an unconventional format, but it is hoped that it will make the volume useful to a wider audience than might otherwise be the case.

On the subject of acknowledgments I will be brief. Stan Wallack and John O'Rourke, of the Office of the Secretary, HEW, provided the original incentive for the work, and it was the efforts of the contributing authors that made the volume possible. I am especially indebted to Mrs. Kathy Kliarsky, who managed the preparation of the final manuscript.

John Rafferty
Chief, Economic Analysis Branch
National Center for Health Services
Research

Part I
Issues in Health Manpower
Productivity

Manpower Substitution in Ambulatory Care

Uwe E. Reinhardt and
Kenneth R. Smith*

Introduction

Throughout the past several decades Americans have been greatly concerned over a shortage of medical manpower. Deficits in the physician supply have been forecast, for successive decades, by a number of government commissions and by several health-manpower specialists. Although the capacity of American medical schools has increased substantially during the last ten years—largely with the assistance of federal funds—allegations of an existing or impending "doctor shortage" persist. These predictions are rendered all the more believable by the prospect of a national health insurance system in this country. The introduction of such a system is expected to trigger large increases in the demand for ambulatory care, for it is primarily the provision of that type of care that has hitherto not been fully covered by health insurance. The production of ambulatory care is, of course, relatively physician-intensive, at least under the current organization of medical practice.

The most straightforward response to increases in the demand for ambulatory care would be to increase the supply of physicians in this country, which in turn can be achieved by subsidizing a continued expansion of American medical schools. From the standpoint of policymakers this approach may seem attractive, for it can be implemented with relative ease. The policy does, however, involve a long gestation period between initial policy action and ultimate policy impact. Furthermore, there is always the possibility that in seeking to avoid manpower deficits in the short run one may inadvertently construct excessive medical school capacity for the longer run.

An alternative response to the alleged physician shortage would be to meet the projected deficits with physician substitutes, that is, health manpower with relatively less formal training than is imparted to physicians and yet capable of taking on many of the less complicated medical and clerical tasks physicians have traditionally performed themselves. It is clear that health-manpower substitution of this sort serves to increase the average hourly productivity of

*The authors are, respectively, Associate Professor of Economics and Public Affairs, Princeton University, and Associate Professor of Economics, The University of Wisconsin. They wish to acknowledge the research assistance of Frederick Boness.

3

physicians and, if physicians do not reduce the length of their workweek, their ability to cope with future increases in the demand for ambulatory care. On the other hand, before rushing headlong into this direction, policymakers obviously need fairly accurate information on (1) the extent to which the proposed manpower substitution is in fact *technically feasible*, and (2) the extent to which that substitution, even if technically feasible, can be justified on *economic* grounds. In connection with the second point, one could hardly expect individual medical practitioners to engage in the proposed task delegation if that implied a decline in their annual net income.

The purpose of this chapter is to survey the literature on health-manpower substitution and to formulate, on the basis of that survey, a more coherent picture of the ambulatory-care production process at the microeconomic level. The chapter will be concerned primarily with the *technical feasibility* of health-manpower substitution, and with the productivity gains that appear attainable through this type of substitution. Of course, both research and policy dealing with increasing physician productivity will also have to consider the nature of incentives that will affect the way in which productivity gains will be allocated; some thoughts along those lines will appear in the concluding section of this chapter, although the topic is dealt with more extensively in another chapter.

Chapter 1 provides a brief review of the theory of production, offered here to highlight different approaches that have been taken to the question of manpower-productivity and substitution. It describes the institutional setting and the various types of health-manpower among whom substitution may be technically feasible and discusses the problem of defining and measuring output. The available literature on the health-care production process is reviewed. We then use pediatric care to illustrate how the available information on one specialty can be synthesized into an overall production function for that type of facility. Finally, we suggest areas for future research.

The Analytical Framework for Production Analyses

The purpose of this section is to indicate briefly (1) the alternative ways in which the production of any good or service can be specified for analytic purposes, and (2) the alternative methods that can be used to estimate empirical values for the parameters thought to characterize the production process. For purposes of that discussion, it will be convenient to assume initially that there exist unambiguous measures of output and inputs for the productive activity under consideration. The difficulty of devising such measures for the content of ambulatory-care production will then be discussed in the next section.

Characterization of the Production Process

It is frequently possible to produce a given rate of output of some good or service with a variety of different combinations of productive inputs. Each particular input combination may be thought of as a distinct technological process or activity, and for each process one can describe the relation between inputs and output by the set of equations

$$L_j = a_j(Q) \cdot Q \qquad j = 1, 2, \ldots, n \qquad (1.1)$$

where L_j denotes the number of units of the jth input required to produce Q units of output, and $a_j(Q)$ is the minimum number of units of the jth required to produce one unit of output if output is being produced at the rate Q. In some production processes the input-output coefficient a_j varies systematically with the rate of production. If each a_j decreases with increases in Q, the process is subject to decreasing returns to scale. For the bulk of production processes, the most plausible assumption is that a_j is constant over all rates of output, i.e., that the production process is subject to constant returns to scale.[1] For the sake of simplicity, we shall make that assumption henceforth, and therefore refer to a $a_j(Q)$ simply as a_j.

It bears repeating that the input coefficients a_j represent the minimum amount of the jth factor required to produce one unit of output: the set of inputs L_j specified in (1.1) is the technically most efficient bundle of inputs to produce Q units of output with the particular technological process under consideration. There may be more than one technical process capable of producing a given rate of output, and then there will be as many distinct technically efficient input combinations as there are distinct production processes. In Figure 1-1 it is assumed that two inputs are transformed into one output, and that this can be done with at least two processes. Process 1 requires at least a_1 of input 1 and a_2 of input 2 to produce one unit of output. The corresponding figures for process 2 are a_2' and a_2', respectively. Both the combinations (a_1, a_2) and (a_1', a_2') are technically efficient in their own right. On the other hand, the combination $(1.5a_1, 1.5a_2)$, if used to produce only one unit of output with production process 1, is technically inefficient, as would be the combination $(1.5a_1', 1.5a_2')$ if used to produce one unit of output with process 2.

Which of the two production processes is optimal in an economic sense, i.e., economically most efficient, is another matter. If the prices of the two inputs are known, one can calculate the production cost per unit of output, and the economically most efficient production process is that resulting in the lowest unit production cost.

Figure 1-1 may also be used to illustrate the distinction between overall

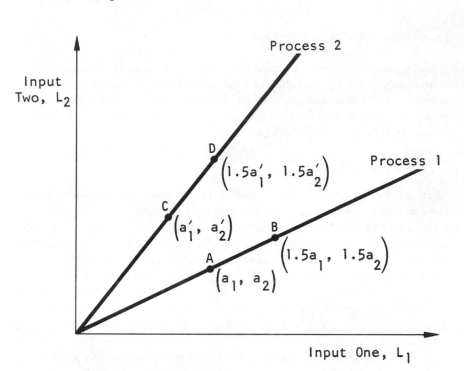

Figure 1-1. Transforming Two Inputs into One Output

productivity gains and gains in the productivity of a particular input, two concepts which are repeatedly confused in the literature. Suppose, for example, that a producer uses technical process 1 in Figure 1-2, but that because of technical inefficiency (e.g., improper plant layout) input combination B is used to produce one unit of output. If the producer succeeds in reorganizing the production process so that one unit of output can be produced with input combination A, then an overall productivity gain has been achieved. The average output for both inputs 1 and 2 has increased. If, on the other hand, the producer's initial position is input combination A and he moves to combination C, then the average productivity of input 1 has been increased though at the expense of the average productivity of input 2 (whose productivity has decreased from $1a_2$ to $1a_2'$). Whether the productivity gain for input 1 is worth "buying" depends on which of the two input combinations is economically most efficient. The proposition that paramedical manpower should be substituted for medical manpower in ambulatory-care production thus is premised on the supposition that such care is currently being produced with economically inefficient production processes.

The arguments made with the aid of Figure 1-1 can be readily generalized to any number of inputs and to any number of processes. If there are n inputs, each

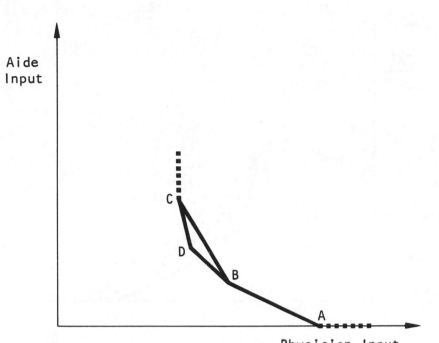

Figure 1-2. Physician Input vs. Aide Input

particular process is characterized by its corresponding set of technically efficient input-output coefficients $(a_1, a_2, \ldots, a_n)$, which indicate the minimum amount of each input required to produce one unit of output. Empirically, the objective is then to identify all the alternative technical "processes" that can, in principle, be used to produce given rates of output. Once these processes have been enumerated, one can then approach the problem of identifying the economically most efficient "process." The entire set of available "processes," properly described, may be referred to as "the production function."

The traditional notion of the production function presupposes that the inputs are continuously substitutable for each other. The model of production outlined above regards each process as inflexible with respect to the ratios among factor inputs and process outputs. Process substitution plays a role analogous to that of factor substitution in the traditional theory. Furthermore, it is assumed that the number of processes available is finite. Thus, it should be possible to catalog all the available alternatives.

The slope of the line segment between two processes (Figure 1-3) represents the rate at which one input must substitute for the other in producing a given amount of medical care. At a point where only one process is being employed, the rate of technical substitution differs according to whether we consider

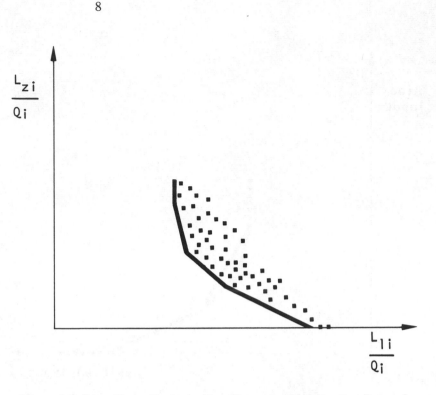

Figure 1-3. Line Slope Between Two Processes Representing Rate of Input Substitution

substituting physician input for that of aides or aide input for that of physicians.[2]

Between any two adjacent processes, it may be possible to identify a third process that uses less of each input than their linear combination. If, for example, process D were introduced, the line segment between B and C would be replaced by line segments BD and DC as in Figure 1-3. As the number of processes increase without limit, line segments shrink toward zero length; there will be an infinite set of processes each contributing one point to the equal product curve. If, in addition, the rate of technical substitution varies continuously, we will have the smooth curve of the traditional production function presentation.

Thus, there is a correspondence between the "process" of "activity" analysis described above and the more traditional analyses based on continuous production functions of the general form

$$q = f(L_1, L_2, \ldots, L_n)$$

(1.2)

where q is thought to be the maximum rate of output attainable with a given input combination $(L_1, L_2, \ldots, L_n)$. In an analysis based on continuous production functions of this sort, one envisages the firm as choosing not among alternative "processes" or "activities," but instead as choosing, for any given rate of output, rates of input utilization.[3]

Alternative Methods of Estimating
Empirical Input-Output Relationships

With a sufficiently large sample of production units using a wide range of technical "processes" and operating at different rates of output, it may be possible to estimate the input-output coefficients of the set of Equations (1.1) or the parameters of the production function (1.2) on the basis of the observed rates of input and output.

The most straightforward estimation method in connection with the activity-analysis approach (i.e., estimation via Equation (1.1)) is probably direct observation of the precise production process. If the sample is varied enough, one can hopefully distinguish among alternative "processes" and identify their empirically relevant range. The main shortcoming of estimating the input-output coefficients a_j on the basis of the actual activities of operating units is that one has no assurance that the units being observed operate the "process" they have chosen in a technically efficient manner. One may therefore fail to identify the technically efficient set of coefficients corresponding to a particular production "process." One way to overcome this might be to base the estimates only on the more efficient production units in the sample. This approach is illustrated in Figure 1-1, where it is assumed that two inputs are used to produce one output, and that each technical process is characterized by constant returns to scale. On these assumptions, each production unit in the sample can be identified by the point $(L_{1i}/Q_i, L_{2i}/Q_i)$ where subscript i denotes the individual producer unit, L_{1i} and L_{2i} are the input rates actually used by unit "i" and Q_i is that unit's rate of output. The set of firms in the sample can then be depicted as a set of points as in Figure 1-3.

It is clear that one would wish to base the estimate of the input-output coefficients a_j for alternative processes only on those observations that lie on the convex enclosure LL in Figure 1-3. Firms observed to fall into that enclosure are the relatively efficient firms in the sample, and the enclosure itself may be viewed as an approximation to the efficient production function being sought. If all the firms in the sample are to a large degree technically inefficient, then one simply cannot use the sample to identify the technically efficient set of production "processes." For a two-input production process, that enclosure can be identified visually.[4] For production processes with more than two inputs, say with n inputs, the technically efficient firms will all lie on the convex hull around the set of points ($L_{1i}/Q, \ldots, L_{ni}/Q_i$), $i = 1, 2, \ldots, k$ representing the k firms in one's sample. The facets of this convex hull can be identified with the aid of straightforward linear-programming techniques.[5] All that is required is that the points lying on the convex hull are not subject to large errors of observation.

Continuous production functions such as Equation (1.2) may be estimated statistically—via multiple regression techniques—on the basis of observed input-output combinations ($Q_i, L_{1i}, \ldots, L_{ni}$) for a cross-section of firms. Again, one necessary condition for the identification of the production function is that there be sufficient interfirm variation in the observed input-output rates. But even if that condition is satisfied, several vexing statistical problems remain.

First, the production function to be identified is a relationship indicating the maximum rates of output attainable with alternative combinations of inputs. With some degree of luck, some firms in the sample will actually succeed in achieving the maximum rate of output attainable, in principle, for the particular input combinations they use; the great majority are likely to be less than fully technically efficient. Standard multiple regression techniques, however, determine the parameters of the empirical production function so that the deviations of the actual from the predicted rates of output (the residuals) sum to zero. It follows that one obtains, at best, an average production function instead of the locus of technically efficient input-output combinations. This average is simply a statistical summary of the experience of the firms in the sample.

If the objective is to predict the amount of output that can on average be obtained with given input combinations, then an average production function is more useful than the hypothetical one, because the former reflects the real world. If the objective is to obtain information on the marginal products that can, under ideal conditions, be obtained from an increment in the use of one input then the average production function will yield a valid answer only if, at any rate of input for that factor, its slope is the same as that of the hypothetical function, for the slope of the line is a measure of the marginal product. This condition may be approximately met if, for any input combination, the average absolute difference between the ideal output corresponding to that input combination and the actual, observed rate of output is the same for all input combinations. On the other hand, if the firms deviate from the ideal output rate by an equal percentage of all input combinations, then the empirical production function will tend to understate the hypothetical marginal (incremental) productivity of the inputs.

A second major problem that is encountered in empirical production function research is the so-called least-squares regression bias. Consider, once again, the technology referred to above, and suppose that the firms are profit maximizers in competitive markets. It can be shown that under these conditions firms that are relatively more efficient, technically, than others will tend to employ more of the input than will the relatively less efficient ones. This situation may be described analytically by assuming that there exists a second productive input loosely labelled "managerial ability." Suppose now that, in terms of the value of M, the firms fall into three distinct groups, those with medium ability, those with superior ability, and those with inferior ability. In this situation, the observed input-output combinations are likely to form three clusters, with each cluster corresponding to a distinct one input—one output production function. The estimated production function will be a different curve passing through all three clusters in a way that minimized the sum of the squared deviation of the sample points. This line clearly attributes to input L a marginal productivity for greater than the rate that could actually be achieved even by the relatively most efficient firms. In other words, there is a tendency to overestimate the true marginal productivity of individual inputs.

This bias can obviously be quite serious. The question remains, however, how large the bias is likely to be in actual fact in the context of medical practice. It is likely to be most severe in cases where the firms are profit maximizers or, at least, cost minimizers. If the firms choose their rate of input usage largely without reference to either objective, then the strong positive correlation between technical efficiency (managerial ability) and the rate of input usage is not likely to be present.[6] In that case, the observations need not form distinct clusters but instead are likely to be more evenly distributed about some average line whose slope is itself some average of the three individual production function lines. Although there may still be some estimation bias, it is likely to be less severe. The latter situation may be more descriptive of ambulatory-care production than is the assumption of profit maximization or cost minimization.

One further difficulty with the continuous-production-function approach is that any attempt to estimate a continuous (average) production function requires the specification of an algebraic form of this function prior to estimation. This a priori specification must be developed with great care, since the mathematical properties of the selected function alone can easily predetermine the economic implications of the empirical estimates. Clearly, the selected specification must not impose more substitutability among the various types of medical workers than actually exists, or force the estimated function to suggest forever increasing rates of marginal productivity.

Definition of Inputs and Output
in Ambulatory Care

Any attempt to infer the input-output coefficients of the production function for ambulatory care from observations on a cross-section sample of health-care providers must proceed on the assumption that the definitions of inputs and output used in the analysis are valid for all providers in the sample. Broadly speaking, the output from a medical practice may be defined as the "management of a set of medical conditions," but to make that definition operational it must be translated into some measurable equivalent. In this translation, the specified unit of output must not vary systematically (in terms of its composition) with the configuration of inputs being used. If this condition is not satisfied, differences in the observed input combinations may reflect either the substitution of one factor for another in the production of a common output, or the use of different input combinations in the production of different types of output. In the production analyses being considered here, interest centers exclusively on factor substitution, and it is therefore crucial that inputs and output be defined in reasonably homogeneous units.

The Definition and Measurement
of Ambulatory-Care Output

The ultimate objective of the medical-care industry may be thought to be "good health," and such an approach to output measurement is often advocated in the health industry literature. However, in the health industry (as well as in other industries in which the use of such a measurement notion might be considered) factors other than medical services go into the production of "health," and it is difficult to specify the "health" production processes with sufficient accuracy to derive from these specifications operationally meaningful definitions of output. A more reasonable approach is to treat output from the industry as an intermediary good, and to evaluate the performance of these industries in terms of these goods. In the context of health-care production, output should thus be defined in terms of the set of "medical conditions managed" or in terms of the set of medical services actually delivered by health-care providers, regardless of their ultimate impact on the recipients' health status. That approach has been taken in virtually all previous work on the health-care production process at the microeconomic level.

In developing the proposed definition of ambulatory-care output, it is useful first to classify provider facilities by subgroups, each characterized by a homogeneous mix of medical cases treated. In specifying outpatient production functions, the following categorization suggests itself: Family Practice (GPs), Internal Medicine, Pediatrics, OBG Specialists, and General Surgery. A rough calculation, using average visits per week, a 48-week work year, and the number of physicians of each type who would service a population of 100,000 (determined from national ratios) shows that Internists, Pediatricians, OBG Specialists, and GPs produce approximately 350,000 of the 425,000 outpatient visits demanded by such a population. This calculation, plus the fact that there is a dearth of literature on the office practices of other types of medical specialists, strongly argues for concentrating the search for manpower substitution opportunities in these five specialities.

The common approach in prior health-care research has been to measure "conditions managed" or "services delivered" by ambulatory facilities in terms of patient visits. Where appropriate information is available, this measure can be adjusted for difference in case complexity. Not infrequently, however, researchers have proceeded on the assumption that case-mix (within a given medical specialty) is constant over time or over different providers, so that the visit measure is thus used as an index of output. If this condition is not satisfied, then an attempt should be made to classify visits by major diagnostic categories: the opportunities for substitition among medical inputs—particularly between physicians and paramedical aids—is likely to vary considerably with the type of case being treated. Should this breakdown of the visit data be necessary—i.e., should one detect considerable interpractice variation in the mix of cases treated even within a given medical specialty—then it may be desirable to proceed in terms of an activity-analysis framework rather than in terms of continuous production functions.

Even for a given mix of cases, however, health providers have some leeway in determining the number of visits generated per management of a medical condition. Thus, it would be preferable to measure output from a provider facility by the number of conditions managed (adjusted for case mix) rather than by visits. In that approach, the "number of visits" would be treated as one input in the "medical conditions managed" production function, and one would consider possibilities of technical substitution between other medical inputs and patient visits.

The difficulty with defining output as "conditions managed," or even as "number of patients treated," is that data on these variables are less available than data on "patient visits." Further, it is not obvious that much information is actually lost by using patient visits as the output measure. If the technical opportunities for substitution among various types of health personnel (or among different types of delivery organizations) is largely relative to the technical opportunities of varying the number of visits required to manage a particular medical condition, then the loss of information from proceeding in terms of patient visits will not be great. It is a problem on which further empirical insights are needed.

The Definition and Measurement of Inputs in Ambulatory-Care Production

As suggested above, it is convenient here to view the providers of ambulatory care as firms that purchase or hire productive factors and convert these into medical output. These productive factors include:

1. The time of physicians.
2. The time of auxiliary personnel.

3. The drugs and medical supplies used in treatments.
4. The office space and medical equipment used by the providers (referred to by the generic term "capital").

The list should also include the patient's own time, although that input has typically been omitted because of unavailability of the required data. Since interest here centers on opportunities for substitution of auxiliary personnel for the physician's time, and for substitution among the various types of auxiliaries, we will not deal with the interesting question of the potential for substitution of medical supplies or capital for any or all types of health-manpower.

Within the category of "auxiliary personnel" one should distinguish further among the following types of assistants:

1. Intermediate-level health workers; physician extenders such as the physician assistant, Medex, pediatric nurse practitioners, family nurse practitioners, and nurse midwives.
2. Allied health workers; traditional medical aides such as the Registered Nurse, licensed practical nurses, and medical assistants.
3. Medical technicians, such as X-ray and laboratory technicians.
4. Nonmedical assistants, such as clerical and administrative personnel.

Just as in the case of output definition, the breakdown of auxiliary health-manpower must be made in units that are homogeneous across health-care providers. The precise meaning of homogeneity in this context is, however, itself a problem. Homogeneity could be defined, for example, with reference to the type of training received by paramedical aides. On that basis, the categorization proposed above is probably not suitable because, as Greenfield (1969) has shown, the traditional types of allied health manpower represent a rather wide range of educational attainment. The category of "allied health workers" is thought to include allied health professionals, allied health technicians, and allied health assistants. Allied health professionals (e.g., registered nurses) have typically attained a baccalaureate and often a master's degree; allied health technicians have typically been trained at the vocational school level; allied health assistants often have only a high school education, and have typically been trained on the job as far as health-care delivery is concerned.

With the exception of some of the technicians, we have grouped most of these three types of manpower into the single category "allied health worker," and the question arises as to the legitimacy of treating a registered nurse as similar to a medical assistant, who has much less formal training, and the answer depends on the ways in which the two types of personnel are typically used by the providers. If the RN is used by physicians in essentially the same way as a technician or assistant, then (from the standpoint of production theory) these types of manpower may be treated as the same. Similarly, if a "physician extender" with roughly the same amount of formal training as a registered nurse is used by physicians in a way that differs noticeably from the use to which RNs are put, the two types of manpower should be viewed as distinct categories. Whether the categorization proposed above is appropriate for the purpose at hand is therefore an empirical question. As will be argued below, all available evidence suggests that our classification is, in fact, appropriate.

Prior Research on Health
Manpower Substitution

This section will focus on the literature reflecting the three distinct approaches that have been taken in this field:

1. Descriptions of task delegation, and of the various roles auxiliary personnel can or might play.
2. Estimates of continuous production functions, such as shown in Equation (1.2).
3. Identification of distinct and alternative "technical processes" that can be used to produce given types of output (with processes being defined as in Equation (1.1) and the identification of the most efficient combination of inputs through activity analysis.

Descriptive Studies

Typical examples of descriptive studies are Yankauer, Connelly, and Feldman (1970), Patterson and Bergman (1969), and some of the reports issued periodically in the fortnightly *Medical Economics.* These are usually based on data from mailed questionnaires or through direct observation of the activities within a small set of practices. The results have usually been presented in tabular form or prose, and interpreted at a very general level. The authors of the studies have not typically sought to evaluate the data in terms of rigorous models capable of controlling for interactions among variables, although the cross-tabulations are sometimes designed to indicate such interactions. These descriptive studies constitute a valuable source of background material for more rigorous analysis, yield insight into the institutional setting within which ambulatory care is produced, and often indicate rough magnitudes of the effect of manpower substitution on physician productivity; we shall therefore draw on these studies below. But, many of the studies are based on very small samples, statistical significance of the results is often not reported, and it is difficult to incorporate the results in health-manpower forecasting models of the sort alluded to in the introduction of this chapter.

Estimates of Continuous Production
Functions

The empirical production-function estimates published to date have been based on mail-questionnaire survey data, [Maurizi (1967), and Reinhardt (1970)], or on direct observation of a small number of practices [Boaz (1972), and Kovner (1968)]. Output in these studies has usually been measured by rates of patient visits (sometimes adjusted for case mix), annual gross billings, or a weighted average of services produced, with the weights being furnished by relative value scales [Kovner (1968)]. Inputs have included the physician's own time, indices of capital equipment used (depreciation, or the number of examination rooms used), and the full-time equivalents of various types of paramedical and clerical assistants. The unit of analysis has typically been the individual provider facility.

The merit of statistical production function estimates is that the user is given some idea of the statistical significance of estimated parameters, and that they constitute parametric estimates that can be directly incorporated into wider health-manpower forecasting models. The estimates also enable one to calculate the marginal productivity of individual inputs and the optimal combinations of inputs corresponding to given rates of output and given input prices. Finally, to the extent that the estimated functions can be taken as unbiased, they can be used as baselines for evaluating the technical and economic efficiency of individual provider facilities.

One stringent requirement of this approach is specification of the mathematical form of the function to be estimated prior to estimation. This specification must be made with care, as the mathematical properties of the selected function can predetermine the economic implication of the empirical estimate. This problem is exemplified by Kovner's estimate of a production function for large group medical practices in Los Angeles.[7]

$$Y = 6.6(GP) + 0.11(SP)^2 + 0.31(LABT)^2 + \qquad (1.3)$$
$$0.86(XRAY)^2 + 0.02(CL)^2 + 0.008(KHF)^2$$
$$- 0.007(RN)^2 - 0.014(LVN)^2 - 0.90(ADM)^2.$$

On the basis of his best estimate, Kovner comes to the conclusion that, with the exception of general practitioners, additional inputs of personnel into the practice (with all other inputs being held constant) will yield ever increasing increments in output—and furthermore, that the tradeoff curves (isoquants) between any two types of manpower for given rates of output are concave to the origin. If this were the case, then, for any two inputs, the economically most efficient input combination would include positive amounts of only one factor and zero input of the other. These conclusions therefore conflict with prior knowledge of the ambulatory-care production process. In fact, they are completely predetermined by the algebraic form of the production function used—a second order polynomial with the first order terms omitted for all but the GP input. Such a function will inevitably lead to rather strange empirical estimates.

In his estimates of production functions for private medical practices in the United States, Reinhardt (1970) has specified a function that is more flexible and would appear to be more realistic than that posited by Kovner. Reinhardt's specification:

1. Permits positive rates of output to occur even when the input of aides is zero (the physician can operate his practice without any auxiliary personnel whatsoever).
2. Presupposes that positive rates of capital and physician time input are required to obtain positive rates of patient visits.
3. Permits both increasing and decreasing marginal productivity over the relevant range.
4. Permits both the degree of returns to scale and the elasticity of substitution between factors to vary over the production surface.

The functional form incorporating these characteristics is a modified Cobb-Douglas:

$$Q_t = A \sum_i \left(x_{it}^{a_i} e^{-b_i x_{it}} \right) \cdot e^{\sum_j c_j L_{jt}} -d \left[\sum_j L_{jt} \right]^2 + \sum_s m_s D_{st} \cdot U_t$$

where T denotes the individual physician, and where

Q_t = the physician's weekly volume of patient visits

x_{1t} = H_t, the number of strictly practice-related hours the physician works per week

x_{2t} = K_t, the index of capital usage

L_{1t} = RN_t, the number of registered nurses per physician

L_{2t} = TE_t, the number of medical technicians per physician

L_{3t} = OA_t, the number of office aides per physician

D_{st}, $s = 1, 2, \ldots, n$, is a set of variables further characterizing the physician

and where U_t is a multiplicative error term. The coefficients, based on weekly office visits, were estimated for general practitioners and for pediatricians, OBG specialists, and internists. The estimates for these specialists turned out to be not strikingly different from the GP function.

Two aspects of these estimates are of particular interest here. First, the employment of auxiliary personnel seems to have a pronounced, positive effect on the productivity (average weekly visit rate) of physicians: there is reason to believe that substantial opportunities to increase the physician's productivity through health-manpower substitution do exist. Second, the relative magnitudes of the estimated coefficients for the individual types of aides suggest that, at the margin, each type of aide contributes roughly the same to the physician's productivity. There are, of course, limits to this manpower substitution. The estimated relationship between weekly office visits and the number of aides employed per physician, with physician input held at a constant 50 hours per week, indicates that there comes a point (after about the fifth aide) where further additions to the physician's auxiliary staff add nothing positive to his visit rate. The curves clearly indicate that additions of more than five aides to the physician's practice do not allow further reductions in his own input. The physician is clearly a limiting factor in the production process.

How far the substitution process should be pushed for a given rate of output depends, of course, on the relative value of the physician's own time and the cost of hiring aides. Using an estimated value of physician time of $17 per hour and a weekly wage rate for aides of $100, Reinhardt calculates an optimal level of aide input of 3.7. Since the observed sample average is 1.96, the estimates suggest that that "average" physician could profitably double the present size of his office staff, thereby increasing his output per hour by approximately 20 to 25 percent. The optimum aide input would be higher still if a value greater than $17 per hour is assigned to the physician's own time.

There are several possible explanations for this large deviation from profit maximizing behavior on the part of physicians: individual physicians may not be aware of the profit potential inherent in manpower substitution, they may be fearful that extensive task delegation may violate the legal statutes governing the practice of medicine, or may fear it will increase the probability of malpractice suits even if the quality of the services does not diminish. There are also psychic costs which physicians may associate with the maintenance of a large staff. But, it is also conceivable that the apparently paradoxical behavior of physicians can be explained by a least squares bias in the estimated production function (as discussed above): statistical estimation of ambulatory-care production functions has typically proceeded on the assumption that the degree of "technical efficiency" does not vary systematically with the rates of inputs used by the provider facilities in the sample; it is, however, possible that the utilization of paramedical aides by physicians is positively related to (a) the effectiveness with which they are able to utilize aides (delegate tasks) once the aides are hired, and (b) the effectiveness with which physicians use their own time.

With regard to the first point, consider a situation in which the only medical inputs are physicians and aides and assume that each practice has the same amount of physician time available. Suppose further that all physicians fall in one of two groups regarding their knowledge of how to utilize aides (their degree of technical efficiency) and that the true production functions for these two groups are given by $H(A)$ and $L(A)$ respectively. The total product curves for these two groups are illustrated in Figure 1-4. Given the relative price of aides, the efficient physician will utilize more aides than the inefficient physician, even when both are making the optimal (cost minimizing or profit maximizing) input choice relative to their own technical efficiency. The function derived from a least-square estimate is likely to look like the dotted line. However, it cannot be concluded from this estimate that producers are utilizing too few aides, given their own perception of the technological opportunites for manpower substitution.

With regard to the second point, the question of how well the physician is able to utilize his own time, physicians vary substantially with respect to the time they take to care for particular types of patients. The more acumen a physician has in managing his own time, the faster he will be able to care for each patient, and with a given amount of his own time, and without extensive delegation of medical activities, some physicians will care for more patients per week than others. Clearly, then, if there are a more or less constant set of clerical and housekeeping activities per patient, the physician who produces more patient visits per week will tend to hire more aides to perform the derivative ancillary chores. This is not a case in which more aides allow the physician to

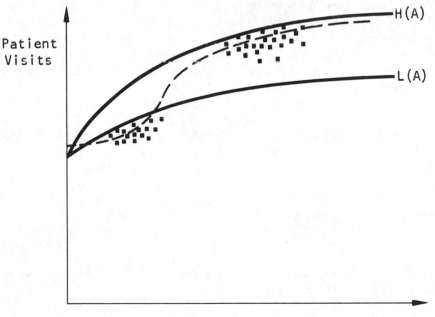

Figure 1-4. Total Product Curves for Aide Utilization by Physicians

produce more visits, but rather a case where the production of more visits requires the presence of more aides.

The conclusion emerging from the foregoing discussion is that, in order to determine the opportunities for technical substitution among types of health-manpower, it behooves us to examine carefully the role each type of manpower can play in the management of medical conditions. This brings us to the subject of task and activity analysis.

Activity Analyses of
Ambulatory-Care Production

As was indicated above, the alternative to characterizing the production of ambulatory care in terms of continuous production functions is to describe it in terms of sets of distinct "technical processes" that can be used to produce given medical treatments. Smith, Miller, and Golladay (1972) have based their analysis of medical practices on that approach.[8]

The authors were able to identify about 200 distinct techniques ("processes") that can be used to produce a total of 41 different medical managements.[9] However, the "processes" identified do not necessarily reveal the technically efficient production function: the manpower combination per unit of output identified for a given "process" is not necessarily the minimum of each input technically required to produce that unit of output; instead, just as in the case of a production function estimate, the authors' empirical characterization of the ambulatory-care production processes merely reflects the actual collective experience of the medical practices in their sample.

Table 1-1 presents the estimates of the alternative combinations of three types of health manpower (in hours per week) that could be used to produce a total of 120 patient visits per week. The listed staffing requirements refer to medical contact time with patients only, so that 28 hours of physician time represents a full-time commitment on the part of the physician. His remaining office hours would be devoted to noncontact activities.

The 120 patient visits underlying Table 1-1 represent a given mix of medical managements—in particular, the selected 41 medical conditions in given propor-

Table 1-1
Staffing Patterns for Managing 120 Particular Patient Visits per Week (Total Hours of Medical Contact Time)

Doctor	26.0	23.2	19.7	18.2	17.25	15.33	11.5	10.6
Med. asst./RN/LPN	1.0	4.0	7.7	9.0	9.0	9.0	8.6	8.7
Physician asst.	0	0	0	0	1.1	3.1	7.1	8.4

Source: Smith, Miller, and Golladay (1972), p. 221.

tions. A different mix of cases would alter the manpower-substitution possibilities for 120 patient visits. It was assumed that in the treatment of some medical conditions (e.g., sore throats) the physician assistant completely substitutes for the physician, while essentially no substitution takes place for more complicated cases, such as heart disease. If the percentage of patients with sore throats increases relative to the percentage of patients with heart ailments, there will be correspondingly greater opportunities to substitute paramedical for medical manpower, given a fixed number of patient visits.

However, it should be noted that the empirical basis for these estimates was crude. For one thing, they found that, first, total medical contact time by all personnel in managing a medical condition was found not to depend on the extent of delegation, which conflicts with a number of other studies in which a greater total time was found to be required when the assistant performs the service than when it is performed by the physician. Second, the study was based on a particularly small number of practices. Further studies along these lines, however, would refine our understanding of the delegation process.

Zeckhauser and Eliastam (1974) also have analyzed the opportunities for utilizing a physician's assistant in an activity-analysis framework. The authors defined two "techniques" or "processes" for producing each element in a vector of medical services: one "process" was defined by a combination of inputs excluding physician assistants, and the other by a combination that did not. The data were obtained from a time-utilization study of a major urban health center producing 60,000 patient visits per year. These visits were provided primarily by internists (25,000) and pediatricians (30,000).

The "technology" without a physician assistant was described by fixed proportions in physician input and a general input called "support," the latter including the physician's traditional auxiliary personnel. The physician assistant is assumed to substitute for the physician. In addition, there may be alterations in the levels of support input. The authors show combinations of physician assistants and support that could substitute for various proportions of a unit of physician; for example, one physician assistant together with an additional annual support flow costing $5000 would substitute for 40 percent of the physician's time.

The authors fit a constant-elasticity-of-substitution (CES) production function to their data and obtain an estimate of 2.94 for the elasticity of substitution. This a priori specification of the production function is unfortunate, however, for at least two reasons. First, it is improbable that the elasticity of substitution between physicians and physician extenders is constant over the entire range of conceivable physician/physician-assistant ratios. A priori, one would assume that in this type of manpower substitution a point is soon reached at which it will be impossible to substitute further physician-assistant time for the physician's own time. But, even accepting the constancy of the elasticity coefficient, it is not likely to be as high as 2.94: that level of the coefficient implies that the isoquant between physicians and physician extenders can cut the axes, and, therefore, that a medical practice can make do without any physician input whatsoever.

These shortcomings of the Zeckhauser-Eliastam study notwithstanding, the approach is an interesting way to obtain a continuous-production-function estimate for ambulatory care from a few data points generated through careful, direct observation of a medical practice. In fact, the proposed synthesis of prior research to be discussed presently will be a variant of that general approach.

A Synthesis of Prior Research

The difficulty with using this body of prior empirical research is that, for the most part, the various studies have examined the opportunities for manpower substitution in a partial and, as a result, noncomparable fashion. Each study has focused on a particular type of auxiliary health personnel, either strictly using the traditional types of paramedical assistants, or primarily the physician extender. There has not to date been any attempt to synthesize these independent studies and to fashion from them a coherent picture of the substitution possibilities among all types of health manpower that appear to be technically feasible. In this section such a synthesis is attempted. One objective is to demonstrate the potential for utilizing a series of independent and narrowly-focused studies to develop a more comprehensive understanding of the production process in ambulatory care. Focus here will be limited to pediatric care, but while some of the details may differ slightly among the major types of ambulatory provider facilities, the general picture gleaned from the pediatric research should be representative of other specialties as well.

We will take as a baseline the physician working by himself. Here, the physician would be involved not only in direct patient care but also in clinical support activities (sterilizing or maintaining equipment, ordering drugs, etc.), clerical and administrative activities, and, if done within the practice, X-ray and laboratory procedures. He could initially delegate some support activities to an RN, a medical technician, or even to personnel without formal training. These have, in fact, been traditional functions of an allied health worker in an office practice.

The Role of Traditional Allied
Health Workers (AHWs)

Several specific research findings, when integrated, furnish a reasonably comprehensive picture of the role and function of the traditional allied health worker in the pediatrician's office practice. First, AHWs spend a relatively small percentage of their total working time in direct contact with patients, and, during the time they do spend with patients, they are mostly engaged in purely mechanical and social types of tasks.[10]

Second, as we have noted, Yankauer, Connelly, and Feldman (1970b) found that the amount of delegation of clerical and technical tasks increases as the number of aides per practice increases, but that the amount of direct patient care is not significantly affected by the number of allied health workers.

Third, although Yankauer et al. found that the amount of delegation of technical tasks to an aide is affected by whether or not the aide is an RN, a number of studies have found that the type of aide used has actually little impact on the pattern of delegation. Patterson and Bergman (1969) report that pediatricians use an RN in essentially the same way they do a medical assistant whose training is only six months. Smith, Miller, and Golladay (1972) also observed that, for particular medical services, a practice utilizing an RN would delegate in much the same way as a practice that employed either a medical assistant or an LPN. This suggests that either the aide is being utilized as an assistant to the MD while he is involved in direct patient care or, alternatively, that the aide is performing rather technical (supportive) tasks. This evidence supports the classification of RNs, LPNs, and medical assistants into the one category of "allied health workers." It further explains why it has been found expedient in some training programs to provide RNs (whose medical training has been much more extensive than LPNs and medical assistants) with additional status through a "laying on of hands" exercise, in order to get physicians to increase the extent to which they delegate direct patient care activities to them. The result has been the emergency of the so-called Pediatric Nurse Practitioners, Family Nurse Practitioners, and Nurse Midwives, and a substantial improvement in their utilization.

Fourth, Reinhardt (1970) finds that as the number of aides in the practice increases, the number of patient visits increase even when other factors are controlled. With Reinhardt's approach one is not able to explain precisely *how* the practice workload is being readjusted (i.e., precisely how tasks are delegated) as the number of aides employed increases, but he does observe that the increase in output caused by the addition of the first aide is much the same regardless of the type of aide being hired.

Integrating these factors, the following picture of the allied health worker's role emerges: The traditional allied health worker appears to be limited, for the most part, to nondirect patient care activities, and the amount of substitution of AHW time for physician time in the area of direct patient care has typically been minimal in actual practice. (It should be emphasized that we are discussing here the actual role of the AHW as it emerges from a number of empirical studies and not the potential use of this type of medical manpower.) An important conclusion that follows from this description of the role and function of the AHW, then, is that the AHW's impact on the practice (the amount by which the

AHW increases the output of the practice or, alternatively, the amount by which physician input can be reduced) is virtually unaffected by the particular mix of cases which the practice confronts. This is an interesting and important conclusion, because it suggests that interpractice case-mix variation is not likely to be a source of serious estimation bias in the type of production-function study reported, say, by Reinhardt (1970).

The Role of Physician Extenders

In caring for a patient, the most readily discernible actions of physicians and other health professionals are the performance of tasks. The development of the intermediate level health worker has been based on the idea that an increasing number of these tasks are sufficiently well defined operationally that they can be delegated to the health practitioner. However, in addition to the performance of tasks, the management of a particular medical condition also includes the expertise which attempts to produce for, each specific patient coherent medical care. The existence of such higher level decision procedures, which physicians employ to ensure that the specific combination of tasks responds to the medical needs of each patient, places constraints on feasible patterns of delegation. These higher level decision procedures may be expressed in the form of relatively simple standard operating procedures (in which case substantial delegation would be feasible), or the decision strategy involved may be sophisticated to the point of almost defying articulation (in which case the involvement of a health practitioner would not be feasible).

During the past decade over one-hundred programs have been developed to train various types of physician extenders (also referred to as health practitioners). These programs, predicated on the notion that much of the activity of the practicing physician is highly repetitive and requires less training and clinical expertise than he possesses, vary substantially in the length and type of training, in the type of person selected for training, and in the type of responsibilities for which the practitioner is trained. The more popular types of health practitioners, oriented toward the primary care area, are the physician assistant (PA), the Medex, the pediatric nurse practitioner (PNP), the Child Health Associate, the family nurse practitioner, and the nurse midwife, but there are also a wide variety of specialty assistants.

There can be little doubt that the widespread, efficient utilization of new intermediate-level health workers could have a substantial impact on the productivity of the medical care delivery systems. Yet, it is difficult to determine the potential role of a health practitioner in the medical delivery process on the basis of actual utilization patterns. For many reasons, the empirical evidence need not describe the "potential impact." As Yankauer (1972) has noted, "the constraints, pressures and personal styles of the setting which delivers care are more important determinants of how personnel will be utilized than the generalities of a job description." As a result, we must be very careful in our interpretation of health practitioner impact. The critical nature of the words "widespread" and "efficient" cannot be overemphasized. As indicated in the introduction, we are concerned with the potential efficient use of health practitioners.

Pediatricians have been at the forefront in exploring the potential of task delegation from physicians to "physician extenders." It seems reasonable, therefore, to begin analysis of the impact of the health practitioner by examining the opportunities for substitution between the physician and the new intermediate level health worker in a pediatric practice.

The most common role proposed for a pediatric nurse practitioner (PNP) is that of a substitute for the physician in the area of well infant and well child care. Every study of pediatric practice has found that the pediatrician sees a large number of well patients and spends a significant portion of his time on them. The figures, of course, vary from study to study, but they all suggest that roughly 40 percent of the patients are well and 50 percent of the pediatrician's patient contact time is devoted to well care.

In addition to well child care, another 30 percent of the pediatrician's time is devoted to minor illnesses. These include the common cold, upper respiratory tract infections, ear infections, and gastro-intestinal disorders. In the area of sick child care, the substitution of the PNP's time for that of the physician may involve the delegation of only certain aspect of the sick child routine. For example, the PNP might make a preliminary analysis and order certain types of tests to aid the physician in his diagnosis. Alternatively, if there exist standard clinical procedures it might be possible for the PNP to completely care for some fraction of the patients in this group. The remainder would be referred to the physician as instructed by the standard procedure.

The physician also spends a substantial amount of time on telephone contact. A survey by the American Academy of Family Physicians revealed that "unnecessary phone calls to the doctor" was the single most annoying thing patients do. At least for the part of this activity that takes place during office hours a PNP, by screening out routine calls, can substitute for some physician time.

Finally, the PNP may be regarded in part as an additional allied health worker of the traditional type. However, to the extent that this is a more expensive input than the allied health worker, it would never be economically efficient to use the PNP in this way.

An Integration of Prior Research

We now attempt to quantitatively synthesize the opportunities for substitution between the physician and physician extender in delivering medical care to a representative pediatric population. We take as our norm the number of pediatric visits performed by the physician who is not utilizing a PNP. It should be noted in terms of our discussion of allied health workers that such a physician may still be using assistants. For example, from Reinhardt's (1970) estimates, a pediatrician with two allied health workers (that is, a medical secretary and a medical assistant or LPN) can produce 124 patient visits per week, and, in so doing, will devote 34 hours of his own time to office practice activities. Of course, only part of the physician's total office time is devoted to direct patient care. For purposes of this illustration, we assume that 28 hours a week is patient contact time. In Figure 1-5, point A represents the combination of 34 physician office practice hours that, with two AHWs and without the assistance of any PNP, can deliver care to 124 pediatric patients.

Most studies so far have found that it takes a PNP more than one minute of time to replace one minute of physician time, for two reasons. First, it is necessary for the pediatrician to commit some time to supervise, consult with, and audit the PNP, so that even if the PNP could carry out the procedures in the same amount of time as the physician, all of the physician's time would not be released for other activities. Second, it is likely that the PNP will take more time to perform the actual procedures associated with the care of a well person. If standard procedures are defined for a well child examination, it may be necessary for the PNP to follow these procedures more systematically than the physician; the physician, with his greater expertise and breadth of training, may short-cut these procedures.

Zeckhauser and Eliastam (1974) found that a PNP engaged for a full day (eight hours) in well child care only can replace one half that much time (four hours) of a pediatrician. In an independent study by Charney and Kitzman (1971) it is reported that average time for a well child visit was 12.8 minutes for the physician and 21 minutes for the PNP.[11]

On the basis of this evidence it is reasonable to assume that one PNP can substitute for the 50 percent of the pediatrician's time which he devotes to well child care. Thus, with one PNP the physician could devote 14 fewer hours per week to the practice without a reduction in the number of patients who receive care (Figure 1-5), and so point B represents an alternative combination of physician time and PNP utilization that also allows the practice to provide 124 patient office visits per week.

Further substitutions can only be achieved by involving the PNP in sick child visits. In addition to the large amount of well child care, the pediatrician also devotes a substantial amount of time to minor illnesses. Assessing the rate of substitution involves determining, for a given disease, the amount of physician time saved and the amount of PNP time required to perform the delegated tasks. In gross terms, the PNP might save roughly two or three minutes of physician time for patients with Otitis media, upper respiratory tract diseases, bronchitis, and tonsilitis. This would release two hours of physician time (for 35 patients)

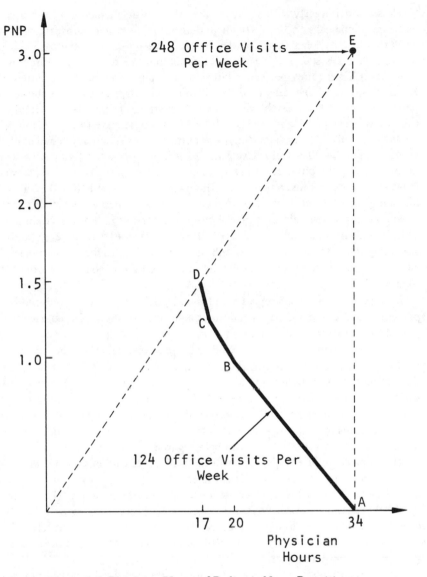

Figure 1-5. Physician Usage of Pediatric Nurse Practitioners

and may involve six hours of PNP input. The result is represented by point *C* in Figure 1-5, where we have assumed that a full-time PNP is equivalent to 30 hours of medical contact time per week. If there existed standard clinical procedures, it might be possible for the PNP to completely care for some fraction of the patients in this group, thereby releasing additional physician time. Unfortunately, the evidence on this point is still rather limited.

Hessel and Haggerty (1968) report that the physician spends 11.9 hours per week on phone calls.[1,2] It is difficult to determine the rate of substitution of the PNP for the physician in telephone contact. We have some evidence on how much time PNPs spend in telephone contact but we do not know how much time the PNP requires per call relative to the physician. In the Charney and Kitzman study, phone calls to the PNP were encouraged and a telephone time period for the PNP was established. The net effect was to increase the number of calls by the group being treated by a PNP-MD team, relative to the calls received by the MD only. At the same time, the number of calls actually handled by the physician fell by 20 percent. Using the 11.9 hours per week figure, this would mean a saving in physician time of slightly more than 2¼ hours per week. However, we do not know how much time was spent by the PNP in handling the remaining calls. It also remains to be determined whether the delegation of telephone contact should take place before or after delegation of sick child care. This would depend on the relative efficiency of the PNP in each activity. Assuming that the delegation of telephone contact follows the delegation of sick child care, it can be represented by the movement from point C to point D in Figure 1-5.

In summary, Figure 1-5 suggests that the physician time can be reduced by 50 percent by the use of 1.5 pediatric nurse practitioners. Of course, if the physician wants to fully utilize the same amount of his own time, then the number of patient visits per period will increase. Holding the pattern of manpower utilization constant, the practice could double in size; in Figure 1-5 this amounts to expanding out along a ray from the origin through point D until we hit the constraint representing the full utilization of the 34 physician hours and the use of three PNPs. Of course, as the practice expands, we assume that the percentages of well care and minor illnesses remain unchanged; thus the same fraction of total practice activity can be delegated.[1,3]

The expansion of the practice will naturally result in an increase in clinical and clerical support activities. Thus more allied health workers will be hired and/or part of the PNP's time will be devoted to these activities. The picture of the PNP presented above was that of a health professional devoted full time to direct patient care. One might speculate that substantial role confusion will be created in the mind of physician, PNP, and patient if they are also used for traditional support activities.

The above analysis has been an attempt to describe the potential impact of a health practitioner in a pediatric office setting. The gains in pediatrics are dramatic primarily because the average pediatrician spends so much of his time in well patient care. In general practice the percentages of well patients is lower. However, the combination of well care and minor illnesses also accounts for a significant part of general practice activity, implying that a substantial part of the practice activity could still be delegated to an assistant.

There is an important qualification that must be made regarding the above presentation. In our description of the opportunities for technical substitution among the physician, the allied health worker, and the physician extender, we have treated all inputs as continuously divisible. In fact, personnel usually must be hired for full-time assignments. Thus, assuming our description of the substitution opportunities is correct, the physician is constrained regarding the particular combinations of health manpower he can actually choose. The fact that he has to fully utilize his personnel may result in the PNP taking on some of the duties of the traditional allied health worker. Actual substitution opportunities will not be as described but will be modified by the constraint of full-time employment.

This qualification lies at the heart of a discussion of economies of scale. There has been considerable debate about whether group practice is more efficient than solo practice in delivering medical care services. While for some time the answer provided to this question was in the affirmative, thus supporting a policy that encouraged group practice, a number of economists have more recently taken a more negative view of the issue. This topic is given more comprehensive treatment in another chapter, but what the above suggests is that an important difference between a small practice and a clinic may be that the clinic has more flexibility in the mix of health manpower it can utilize and in the way the production process is organized. Furthermore, the benefit of this flexibility appears to be more important if medical tasks are delegated to physician extenders than if only nonmedical tasks are delegated to allied health workers. As a result, care must be exercised in interpreting the historical evidence (or lack thereof) on scale economies, since until recently actual experience has been limited to the latter type of delegation. The medical activities of the clinic may also have to be more integrated than is the case in many "group practices"; the latter may be more accurately described as collections of solo practitioners operating under a common roof.[14]

Finally, the amount of substitution and the resulting increase in physician productivity which will actually occur will also be affected by the opportunities to expand the size of the practice. It cannot automatically be assumed that the people who need additional medical care are distributed geographically such that increased productivity of the currently practicing physician can serve this need. If one community has an adequate supply of medical care (that is, enough physicians operating in the traditional mode), physician extenders are not likely to be utilized. On the other hand, a community without a physician would not be able to benefit from a physician extender, even though such a person could respond to the problems for which a majority of medical contacts are initiated.

Clearly, the technical feasibility of manpower substitution is but part of the story. In addition to considerations of technical feasibility, we must also be concerned with (1) the organization of the delivery system—for example, the role of health practitioners as a solution to the problem of access to the system may well be dependent upon the development of a new organization of the medical care delivery system that can better facilitate their use, and (2) the available supplies of health manpower. In addition, we must be especially concerned with the economic incentives faced by the physician who decides how the medical care process is organized, a topic which is dealt with in another chapter of this volume.

Suggested Research

Further concrete information is needed on the extent to which task delegation from medical to paramedical personnel is technically feasible. This information requires further estimation of parameters characterizing the health care production process. In addition, however, it will be necessary to gain further insights also into the production decision process in health-care delivery; a technical potential for health-manpower substitution is of interest only if health-care providers can be induced to exploit the potential economic benefits.

The production-function research already published, along with that which is currently in progress, will, when completed, have exploited the information that can be elicited from physicians via mail-questionnaire. The bulk of that research—as it concerns the question of manpower substitution—involves the estimation of continuous production functions of various forms, with output still measured at a fairly aggregate level (e.g., visits). The information generated by ongoing research will be useful even if it only corroborates existent research results. However, further replication of that research will not be a valuable source of new information.

The logical next step in the analysis of ambulatory-care production will be the procurement of empirical information through *direct observation* of medical practices. Such direct observation may take the form of monitoring the activities within a practice at a fairly general level or, at the other extreme, of following patients through the facility and recording their contacts with various types of health manpower in detailed time-and-motion studies. Direct observation of medical practices can, of course, become enormously expensive, and in launching such research one does well to keep in mind its opportunity costs. On the benefit side, however, the following advantages suggest themselves:

1. Emphasis on direct observation will provide a better understanding of the actual process of health-care production, and, particularly, of the process of task delegation.
2. Direct observation makes it possible to obtain far more refined output measures that can be obtained via mailed questionnaires. The number of visits generated per episode of a given illness can vary considerably among provider facilities, and over time for a given provider facility. Also, the logical extension of existing production—function research is to estimate such functions at the more disaggregate level.

3. Direct observation will substantially reduce the observation errors and sampling biases that beset literally all the variables on which data is obtained via mailed questionnaires.
4. Research findings based on direct observation—in addition to providing a more accurate basis for manpower policy—are also likely to be more useful as guides for individual provider facilities.

With respect to the latter point, research on manpower substitution will be even more useful to individual provider facilities if the stochastic nature of the ambulatory-care production process is explicitly acknowledged in the model. This analytic development will be especially important for models using the activity analysis approach.

So far, the bulk of research on the substitution of paramedical for medical manpower has involved mainly the traditional types of paramedical personnel—registered or licensed practical nurses, medical and X-ray technicians, and clerical personnel. Future research should concentrate more heavily on the role of the physician assistant in task delegation. The term "physician assistant" does not represent manpower of a standard type, but embraces an entire spectrum of different levels of training. Although a good number of evaluation projects on this type of manpower are currently underway, economists have yet to play a major role in such research. If these evaluations are to be incorporated in formal manpower forecasting models, the role of physician assistants must be evaluated in terms of models (i.e., economic models) that are compatible with these forecasting models.

By their very nature, statistical or activity-analysis estimates of production surfaces based on operational data reflect a mixture of the technically feasible and the customarily or legally acceptable. There would be great merit, therefore, in seeking to estimate production functions that are more akin to the so-called engineering production functions sometimes developed for industrial processes. In this effort the economist will, of course, have to team up with experienced, competent, and imaginative medical practitioners. But ultimately it is the direction that will have to be followed in order to estimate efficient rather than average production functions for ambulatory care.

Joint research efforts of economists and medical practitioners will also protect the economist from one error to which he or she is especially vulnerable: the confusion of productivity gains with decreases in the quality of health care delivered. It is assumed by some writers in the health field that the delegation of tasks from medical to paramedical personnel will inevitably proceed at the risk of dilution in the quality of medical care. Economists have so far had to assume this problem away a priori, or instead have sought to control for it in rather crude ways. More information on the relationship between the objective quality of medical services and the extent of task delegation would be a welcome addition to the state of the art in this research area.

We have seen above that almost all research on health manpower substitution' points to the conclusion that the typical provider of ambulatory care—individual practitioners or even group practices or clinics—has not pushed the substitution of paramedical for medical manpower to the extent that is economically desirable. This finding leads one to wonder why the medical profession has so far failed to maximize the returns apparently available to it. Indeed, one can measure the lack of efficiency in this context by an index that is the analogue of the "discrimination index" sometimes employed in analyses of labor-market discrimination. One of the research tasks ahead will be to explain the size of this "discrimination coefficient." We have already suggested some of the factors that might act as deterrents to task delegation—the notion that quality deteriorates with the extent of task delegation, a potential fear of malpractice suits, or perhaps even a simple aversion on the part of the physician to the administrative chores involved in directing a large auxiliary staff. Empirical information on the relative importance of these and still other explanatory factors will be an important input into federal and state health-manpower policy.

Notes

1. Except for a few production processes (such as the storage of liquids), it is reasonable to expect that a doubling of *all* the inputs used in the process should lead to a doubling of the rate of output, Q. If there are increasing returns, they tend to reflect the fact that inputs are not perfectly divisible and are underutilized at low rates of output. If decreasing returns are observed, they are typically the result of a failure to increase *all* inputs in the production process proportionately. The omitted factor is typically something one may refer to as "management."

2. Note that the economically efficient combination of processes can be found by comparing this rate of technical substitution with the relative costs of the two inputs, the latter being the rate at which inputs can be substituted in the market place.

3. As in the process or activity analysis case, these rates of input utilization are determined so that, at the margin, the rate of technical substitution (given by the slope of the equal product curve of Figure 1-4) equals the ratio of input prices.

4. One way to envisage the determination of the enclosure is to imagine that each point in Figure 1-5 is a nail hammered into the coordinate and that one puts a string around the southwest portion of the cluster of nails. The string then forms the convex enclosure and may be viewed as the relatively most efficient production function.

5. For a description of this technique, see Farrell (1957).

6. Reinhardt (1970), Appendix 3.

7. Kovner observed the operations of seven Kaiser Foundation Clinics for a

total of seven days. For each of the 49 observations he obtained information on the man-hours worked by general practitioners, specialists, registered nurses, licensed vocational nurses, laboratory and X-ray technicians, administrative staff, and clerical personnel. Capital input was measured in terms of floor space available at each clinic.

8. Beginning with a compilation of detailed data on the task content of general medical practice, medical student observers recorded the time expended by various health personnel on each of 263 tasks. Insights were thus gained into feasible patterns of task delegation and on the time required by physician and nonphysician personnel to perform each task. The sample included two practices that employed intermediate-level health workers who had graduated from the Duke University Physician Assistant Program.

9. Approximately 80 percent of the patient visits could be classified into one of these services.

10. See Patterson and Bergman (1969), and Silver and Duncan (1971).

11. The 12.8 minutes of physician time per visit is quite consistent with the estimates obtained in other studies; Smith et al. (1972) estimated 14 minutes and Bergman et al. (1966) estimated 13 minutes of physician time per visit.

12. This also includes calls which are handled in other than the office setting.

13. This also assumes that the amount of nonoffice practice activity does not change. If it increases proportionately, then the amount of physician time available for office practice activities falls as the number of patients increases. As a result, the practice expansion may be limited to approximately 55 additional patients, an increase of 44 percent rather than 100 percent. The actual result is likely to be between these two extremes.

14. The implications of these indivisibilities are systematically explored in Golladay, Manser and Smith (1974).

Bibliography

American Nurses Association and the American Academy of Pediatrics Joint Statement of the "Guidelines on Short-Term Continuing Education Programs for Pediatric Nurse Practitioners," *American Journal of Nursing*, Vol. 71:509 (March 1971).

Andrews, P.M., and A. Yankauer, "The Pediatric Nurse," *American Journal of Nursing*, Vol. 73:504 (March 1971).

Bailey, R.M., "Economies of Scale in Medical Practice," in *Empirical Studies in Health Economics*, edited by Herbert E. Klarman. Baltimore: The Johns Hopkins Press, 1970.

Bear, D.V.T., "The Economics of Medical Care," unpublished, March 20, 1963.

Bergman, A.B.; S.W. Dassel; and R.J. Wedgwood, "Time-Motion Study of Practicing Pediatricians," *Pediatrics*, Vol. 38:254 (August 1966).

Bergman, A.B.; J.L. Probstfield; and R.J. Wedgwood, "Performance Analysis in a Pediatric Office," *Journal of Medical Education*, Vol. 42:249 (March 1967).

_____, "Task Identification in Pediatric Practice," *American Journal of the Disabled Child*, Vol. 113:459 (September 1969).

Boaz, R.F., "Manpower Utilization by Subsidized Family Planning Clinics: An Economic Criterion for Determining the Professional Skill Mix," *Journal of Human Resources*, Vol. 2:191-207 (Spring 1972).

Breese, B.B.; F.A. Disney; and W. Talpey, "The Nature of a Small Pediatric Group Practice," *Pediatrics*, Vol. 38:264 (August 1966).

Cassels, Jane, and Harold R. Cohen, "The Introduction of Midwifery in a Prepaid Group Practice," *American Journal of Public Health* Vol. 62:354-360 (March 1972).

Charney, E., and H. Kitzman, "The Child Health Nurse (PNP) in Private Practice," *New England Journal of Medicine*, Vol. 285:1353 (December 9, 1971).

Farrell, M.J., "The Measurement of Productive Efficiency," *The Journal of the Royal Statistical Society*, Vol. 120, Part 3, 1957, pp. 253-281.

Feldman, Marie, "Pediatric Nurse Practitioners' Role in a Large Group Practice," *Hospital Topics*, Vol. 50:62 (March 1972).

Fink, D.; H.J. Malloy; M. Cohen; M.A. Greycloud; and F. Martin, "Effective Patient Care in the Pediatrics Ambulatory Setting: A Study of the Acute Care Clinic," *Pediatrics*, Vol. 43:927-935 (June 1969).

Freeman, John R., "Manpower Analysis for General Medical Practice," Final Report for a contract from BHME-NIH, 1971.

Golladay, F.L.; M.E. Manser; and K.R. Smith, "Scale Economies in the Delivery of Medical Care: A Mixed Integer Programming Analysis of Efficient Manpower Utilization," *The Journal of Human Resources*, Vol. IX, No. 1 (Winter 1974) pp. 50-62.

Greenfield, Harry I., *Allied Health Manpower: Trends and Prospects*. New York: Columbia University Press, 1969.

Hessel, S.J., and R.J. Haggerty, "General Pediatrics: A Study of Practice in the Mid-1960's," *Journal of Pediatrics*, Vol. 73:271 (August 1968).

Kovner, J.W., "A Production Function for Outpatient Medical Facilities," unpublished Ph.D. dissertation, University of California, Los Angeles, 1968.

Maurizi, A., "The Economics of the Dental Profession," unpublished Ph.D. dissertation, Stanford University, 1967.

Morgan, Cynthia A., "How an OB Nurse Specialist Functions," *Hospital Topics* Vol. 50:71-74 (March 1972).

National Advisory Commission, *Report of the Commission of Health Manpower*, Vol. 1:2, November 1967.

Patterson, P.K., and A.B. Bergman, "Time-Motion Study of Six Pediatric Office Assistants," *New England Journal of Medicine*, Vol. 281:771 (October 2, 1969).

Reinhardt, U.E., "An Economic Analysis of Physicians' Practices," unpublished Ph.D. dissertation, Yale University, 1970.

_____ , "Manpower Substitution and Productivity in Medical Practice: Review of Research," *Health Services Research*, pp. 200-27 (Fall 1973).

_____ , "A Production Function for Physicians' Services," *Review of Economics and Statistics*, Vol. 54: 55-66 (February 1972).

Riddick, F.A.; J.B. Bryan; M.I. Gershenson; and A.C. Costello, "Use of Allied Health Professionals in Internists' Offices," *Archives of Internal Medicine*, Vol. 127:924-31 (May 1971).

Schiff, D.W.; C.H. Frazer; and H.C. Walters, "The PNP in the Office of Pediatricians in Private Practice," *Pediatrics*, Vol. 44:62 (July 1969).

Silver, H.K., and B. Duncan, "Time-Motion Study of Pediatric Nurse Practitioners: Comparison with 'Regular' Office Nurses and Pediatricians," *Journal of Pediatrics*, Vol. 79:331 (August 1971).

Simms, N.H.; H.M. Seidel; and R.E. Cooke, "A Structured Approach to the Use of Physician Extenders in Well-Child Evaluations," *Journal of Pediatrics*, Vol. 79:151-63 (July 1971).

Smith, K.R.; M. Miller; and F.L. Golladay, "An Analysis of the Optimal Use of Inputs in the Production of Medical Services," *Journal of Human Resources*, Vol. 7:208-25 (Spring 1972).

Spallone, J.L., "Survey of Ancillary Health Personnel Employed by Doctors of Osteopathic Medicine in Pennsylvania," Hospital Educational and Research Foundation of Pennsylvania, 1968 (mimeographed).

Yankauer, A., "The Outcome and Service Impact of a Pediatric Nurse Practitioner Training Program/Nurse Practitioner Training Outcome," *The American Journal of Public Health*, Vol. 62 (March 1972).

Yankauer, A.; J.P. Connelly; and J.J. Feldman, "Pediatric Practice in the U.S., with Special Attention to Utilization of Allied Health Worker Services," *Pediatrics*, Vol. 45:521 (supplement, March 1970a).

_____ , "Physician Productivity in the Delivery of Ambulatory Pediatric Care," *Medical Care*, Vol. 8:35 (January/February 1970b).

_____ , "Task Performance and Task Delegation in Pediatric Office Practice," *American Journal of Public Health*, Vol. 59:1104 (July 1969).

Yankauer, A.; S.H. Jones; J. Schneider; and L.M. Hellman, "Performance and Delegation of Patient Services by Physicians in Obstetrics-Gynecology," *American Journal of Public Health*, Vol. 61:1545 (August 1971).

Yankauer, A.; J. Schneider; S.H. Jones; L.M. Hellman; and J.J. Feldman, "Physician Output, Productivity and Task Delegation in Obstetrics-Gynecologic Practices in the U.S., *Obstetrics and Gynecology*, Vol. 39:151 (January 1, 1972).

_____ , "Practice of Obstetrics and Gynecology in the U.S.," *Obstetrics and Gynecology*, Vol. 38:800 (November 1971).

Zeckhauser, R., and M. Eliastam, "The Productivity Potential of the Physician Assistant," *The Journal of Human Resources*, Vol. IX, No. 1 (Winter 1974) pp. 95-116.

Productivity and Economies of Scale in Medical Practice

Richard M. Scheffler*

Introduction

The comparison of the productivity and costs of health care services provided by solo medical practice with those provided by group practice has become a topic of increased interest since the Nixon administration has put forward its original proposal on Health Maintenance Organizations; the related questions concerning such matters as economies of scale and the optimal employment of inputs, especially manpower, have thus also been increasingly emphasized. This chapter deals with these latter questions. It begins by setting forth the relevant theoretical concepts, and then reviews and analyzes the pertinent and recent literature; suggestions are then offered for future research.

It will be helpful to first establish the conceptual framework in which productivity and economies of scale are defined. This is done with particular brevity here, since the previous chapter also dealt with these basic relationships, though in a slightly different context. Solo and group medical practices are conceived of here as using technical production processes within which they obtain the maximum quantity of output from any set of inputs. Each practice solves the problem, "for specified quantities of different types of labor, $L_i, \ldots, L_N$, and capital, $K_i, \ldots, K_M$, produce the maximum possible output, S." The quantities of labor and capital are varied over all possible levels, and a "production function" is derived which maps every possible combination of inputs into the maximum attainable output,

$$S = f(L_1, \ldots, L_N, K_1, \ldots, K_M). \tag{2.1}$$

The maximum attainable output for any factor combination will depend on the way in which the practice or firm is organized to combine inputs, i.e., on the process of production the firm uses. The organizational forms or processes of production are probably quite different in solo and group practices, and we therefore represent the types of practice as having different production functions. Let the solo practice production function be (2.1), and let the group function be

*Assistant Professor of Economics and Research Associate in the Health Services Research Center, University of North Carolina, Chapel Hill.

$$G = g(L_1, \ldots, L_N, K_1, \ldots, K_M).$$ (2.2)

The question of productivity in physician's services is then, "If a number of doctors, D, are available, can more output be obtained by having them practice in one or more groups or by installing them in D solo practices." In practice the other inputs to the production process, such as nurses and equipment, are frequently ignored, although their use certainly affects the output of the practice. Let each solo practice produce an output S_i, and let the group output be G. Then the productivity issue is really the direction of the inequality in

$$\frac{G}{D} \begin{array}{c} > \\ < \end{array} \frac{\displaystyle\sum_{i=1}^{L} S_i}{D}.$$ (2.3)

The direction of the inequality indicates which form of organization has a greater output per physician, i.e., in which type of practice physicians are more productive.

Productivity of all inputs together can only be compared if the inputs $L_1, \ldots, L_N, K_1, \ldots, K_M$ and physicians can be combined into one input, X. Ideally the input, X, and output, G or S, should be measured in purely physical terms. Since physical measures for X and G or S are difficult to define meaningfully, researchers ordinarily weigh each input and each output by its price and use a weighted sum of inputs and outputs. The productivity comparison is then

$$\frac{G}{X_G} \begin{array}{c} > \\ < \end{array} \frac{\displaystyle\sum_{i=1}^{D} S_i}{\displaystyle\sum_{i=1}^{D} X_i}$$ (2.4)

where X_i is the weighted sum of inputs for the ith solo practice.

In contrast to the comparison of output from different production functions as is done in productivity analysis, examination of returns to scale consists of comparing the output of different input levels in the same production function: all inputs are varied in the same proportion, and the resulting behavior of output is observed. Mathematically, in the group production function (2.2) each input is multiplied by a constant n. Let the resulting output be

$$mG = g(nL_1, \ldots, nL_N, nK_1, \ldots, nK_M).$$ (2.5)

If $m = n$ output changes in the same proportion as the inputs and the production function g exhibits constant returns to scale; for $m > n$ there are increasing returns to scale, and for $m < n$, decreasing returns.

Now to the problems of how D doctors should practice if the goal is to maximize their output. Assume they are to practice in groups. At the extremes they can work in $D/2$ groups of two, or in one group of D physicians. If there are constant returns to scale, it makes no difference how they practice because all possible group arrangements for D physicians yield the same total output. With increasing returns, all D physicians should practice in one group. With decreasing returns, it would be optimal to have $D/2$ groups of two doctors each.

As stated above, returns to scale depend on the form of the production function and, as in the case of productivity, returns to scale are ideally measured in purely physical terms. Just as with productivity, purely physical units of measurement are usually unavailable, and resort must be made to price-weighted input and output indices. In the case of scale, however, the use of monetary measures has a basis in conventional theory. For any production function which meets well-known regularity conditions and any firm which acts as if it solves any of a variety of optimizing problems,[1] the production functions has a dual cost function. Let the dual cost function for production function (2.2) be

$$C_g = C(G, W_1, \ldots, W_N, r_1, \ldots, r_M).\tag{2.6}$$

C is a "minimum total cost function because it gives the minimum total cost attainable under the production function (2.2) for output level G where input prices for labor and capital are $W_1, \ldots, W_N, r_1, \ldots, r_M$. Except for G, the output measure, the problem of returns to scale can now be defined entirely in terms of monetary variables, C_g and the factor prices. With constant input prices, if there are increasing returns to scale average costs of production must fall as "scale" is increased: output increases faster than the inputs used to produce it, so that

$$\frac{C_g}{G} = \frac{C(G, W_1, \ldots, W_N, r_1, \ldots, r_N)}{G}$$

will fall as output expands.[2] The fall in average cost as output increases is due to economies of scale; thus, an increasing average cost is called diseconomies of scale, and constant average costs indicate no economies of scale. In practice, once again, output and costs are measured in monetary units.

This brief review illustrates an important conceptual difficulty in the literature on productivity and economies of scale: data on solo and group practices obviously cannot be simultaneously used to study both of these theoretical constructs. Either we believe that solo and group practices have the same production functions, and we study economies of scale, or we believe they have different production functions and we study productivity differences between types of practice and economies of scale within group practices. It is also important to keep in mind that output should ideally be measured independently of all input prices. Any study using physician hours or expenditures on care as an output measure, for instance, is liable to consistently produce biases and errors of measurement.

Productivity Measurements and Comparisons

Reder's attempt (1969) to measure productivity of a comprehensive prepaid medical group (similar to an HMO) involves division of the participants of the plan into treatment-need classes, defined by age, sex, and other relevant variables. For each sample person in each class, he calculated the total numbers and corresponding total values of all medical goods and services used during a based year. These expenditures are summed across each class separately, and each sum is divided by the number of people in that respective treatment-need class. What results is the average value of services used by the value per individual for each class. Each person in the plan is now weighted by the value of medical care per individual for his class, and the weighted sum is computed for the entire comprehensive plan. This is Reder's measure of output at a specified quality.[3] The total value of medical inputs for that base year is computed. Similar data is gathered in subsequent years, and changes in deflated value of input per unit of output should measure productivity.[4] In order to guard against artificial gains in productivity which can result from adulteration of the product or use of unmeasured inputs, Reder proposes a "medical care vector" which states the tradeoff—measured subjectively but numerically—between an increase in measured productivity and a decline in quality measured by some proxy.[5]

This methodology is designed to apply to prepaid plans, although it may easily be extended to a fee for service providers.[6] However, it does have weaknesses. The aggregate measure of output in dollar terms precludes the possibility of changes being identified with any specific input.[7] Martin Feldstein (see Reder, 1969) criticizes Reder's "Cost and Insurance" approach because it fails to distinguish between unit price and total expenditures. He complements Reder's approach with a disaggregated description of the physical health benefits produced, but points to a serious difficulty in estimating the extent to which differences in medical care are responsible for differences in the health variable.[8] Productive and efficient medicine may keep some patients alive who have serious chronic illnesses, without returning them to their original health state. Thus, the question arises whether we wish to measure an output of improvements in health status or simply the quantity of services rendered. A true measure of improved health status would probably show lower productivity. For purposes of comparison, of course, it makes no difference which output measure is used if they move together. Finally, any scheme which proposes to measure output as the dollar value of services produced faces the likely prospect that this figure will include something analogous to an "excess profit" for the owners of the group. Even if the physicians own the group, there is no way of separating out what portion of the total physician net revenue results from their role as specialized factors of production and what portion arises because they also play the role of entrepreneurs exploiting a naturally monopolistic market position.

Richard Bailey (1970) has dealt with the problem of measuring productivity using the production function approach.[9] He asserts that a medical group is a multiproduct firm producing sets of outputs (physician services, laboratory work, etc.) and different products within each set (physicians produce some throat exams, general health checkups, etc.). Each product of each set is produced by a particular production process, and each process is represented by a production function.

$$Y_1 = f^1(K_1, \ldots, K_n, L_1, \ldots, L_m)$$

$$\cdot$$
$$\cdot$$
$$\cdot$$

$$Y_x - f^x(K_1, \ldots, K_n, L_1, \ldots, L_m)$$
$$Y_{x+1} = g^1(K_{n+1}, \ldots, K_r, L_{m+1}, L_t)$$

$$\cdot$$
$$\cdot$$
$$\cdot$$

$$Y_{x+2} = g^2(K_{n+1}, \ldots, K_r, L_{m+1}, \ldots, L_t).$$

The production functions may contain the same or different types of inputs. However, Bailey never estimates this production, although some casual empirical evidence is presented.[10]

Although this work is a significant contribution, Bailey appears to omit several important considerations. Throughout the paper he seems to imply that total social costs are the same whether the patient is treated entirely in one visit or is sent scurrying about for his laboratory tests, X-rays, physical exam, etc.

This ignores the added transactions costs which can be measured by the dollar value of extra patient time which is spent in search and in transit. With regard to the production functions, he ignores possible interrelationships between service sets, and gives scant notice to the possibility of joint production. Further, Bailey's notion about separability of these production functions is open to question. It is likely that an output such as laboratory services would be better thought of as an intermediate input in the production process.[11] Hence, a better formulation might be a two or three level production function.

Using the production function approach discussed in the previous chapter, and employing data from two nationwide surveys of self-employed American physicians, Reinhardt (1970), calculates the productivity differences between solo and group physicians. The data used were from a 1965 and 1967 survey conducted by Medical Economies Incorporated. He uses observations on obstetricians-gynecologists and specialists in internal medicine that are in solo and group practice. Multispecialty groups were eliminated because, as seen by Reinhardt, their production process is significantly different from solo and single specialty groups. His assumption is that single-specialty group physicians practice the same kind of medicine as solo physicians, so that he can use patient visits as a homogeneous output measure. The homogeneity assumption is questionable, since case mix differences are quite likely.[12] A further limitation is that his data do not distinguish between the different kinds of aides (nurses, physician assistants, X-ray technicians, etc.) which are used. Thus, these empirical estimates cannot account accurately for the substitution of different types of aides for doctors.

With cross sectional data including three different measures of output (total patient visits which include office, hospital, home visits, office visits alone, and patient billings) as the dependent variable, Reinhardt fits his preselected functional form to the sample data, and finds that "these estimates suggest that, at given levels of practice inputs, physicians in (single-specialty) groups tend to generate between 4.5 and 5.1 percent more patient visits and 5.6 percent more patient billings than do their colleagues in solo practice." These results do, however, depend directly on the appropriateness of the production function specification, which was chosen at least in part so as to allow positive rates of output when the input of aides is zero, and to permit both increasing and decreasing marginal products over the empirically relevant range of inputs. Although this specification therefore seems quite plausible, it is not the only such function which might have fit the data.[13] More important from a theoretical point of view, there is the question of whether the data actually represents points on the true production function.[14] It should be noted that studies which fit preselected production functions can at best provide good historical descriptions. Of course, there is no alternative to preselection at the conceptual level, but empirical tests of the sensitivity of the results to the functional form used would have increased our confidence in these findings.

Kovner (1968), also used the production function approach, applying it to seven Kaiser Foundation Clinics in Los Angeles. He collected data (for seven days) at each clinic on man-hours of labor inputs and on capital, measured in floor space. The Relative Value Scale (RVS) of standard fees in California was used to weigh the medical services produced. Limiting himself to outpatient services, he separated output into (a) office visits, (b) specific diagnostic services, (c) therapeutic services, (d) surgical services, (e) radiological services, (f) laboratory services, and (g) all other services. This attempt to obtain case mix data was a step in the right direction, but Kovner undoubtedly errs in treating medical goods and services as homogeneous. This decision was based on the assumption that the number of RVS units used to produce these outputs are the same, which seems unreasonable since the averages range from 0.1 for nursing visits to 3.5 for physical exams. However, he claims there is no significant difference between the goods and services delivered for various medical conditions.[15] Thus, the results must be qualified by a number of statistical problems. In short, however, Kovner's results indicate that productivity does increase in prepaid groups as the size of the group increases; this point will be discussed in more detail below.

A major contribution of Kovner is his formulation and use of IMPs, "identifiable medical practices." He defines the IMPs as descriptions of the activities of medical personnel. The activities consist of three phases—the examination phase, the information retrieval phase, and the interaction diagnostic phase. Kovner then presents a detailed explanation of the development of the IMP system for outpatient medical services. He also presents comparisons of the IMP system with other output measures, such as number of patient visits or time spent with patient by physician. This suggests that his system is superior on the basis of its level of disaggregation, at least.

Scale Economies

Closely related to the productivity question is that of economies of scale. Scale economies exist if the unit cost of production can be reduced by increasing the level of production and adjusting all inputs; they thus occur in output regions where the marginal costs are less than average costs. The presence or absence of economies of scale is a basic consideration for the comparison of group and solo practices, since the two are directly linked to diverse scales of operation; the topic has thus been the central issue for several recent papers.

Bailey (1968 and 1970) and Newhouse (1973), argue that economies of scale are not achieved by switching from solo to group practice, while Reinhardt (1970) and Kovner (1968), conclude that they do exist. Each bases his argument on a different data set, and each attempts to validate his argument with different tests. Moreover, it should be recalled that a comparison of solo and group data for economies of scale precludes the consideration of differences in productivity.

Bailey bases his conclusions on comparisons of average physician production (in terms of office visits) for a selected sample of internists in the San Francisco area during April 1967. He found constant returns to scale. Income per physician was higher in the larger practice because, he says, these physicians provide extra ancillary services under one roof. Office visits (weighted by type of visit) per physician were the same for solo and clinics, but were less for smaller groups than for clinics. Further, the ratio of paramedical help to physicians rose as group size increased while physician productivity was actually smaller, and total production per physician remained about the same. According to Bailey, the data suggest that the addition of paramedical personnel does not directly affect physician productivity, but may result in substitution of paramedical time for physician time in nonmedical tasks. Bailey's analysis is interesting, though it does have limitations. No attempt is made to standardize the output differences which may exist between the solo and group practice. Furthermore, the data did not permit an examination of the utilization pattern for paramedical personnel by group and nongroup physician. In addition, the type of paramedical aid was not specified.

Newhouse, while agreeing with Bailey that economies of scale are not present, takes a different route, using data from 20 medical practices in Los Angeles which include eleven different physician specialties.[16] He tests an "x-inefficiency hypothesis." This hypothesis states that, as the size of the medical group increases, each ". . . physician is less likely to have to hear the financial consequences of his decision . . ." and he therefore behaves inefficiently. Briefly, the basic empirical model used to test this hypothesis is as follows: the dependent variable, average costs, is measured by average salary costs per office visit excluding salaries for ancillary personnel. It is regressed on the number of office visits, visits squared, and a dummy variable which indicates whether the practice had a cost sharing agreement.[17] The positive and statistically significant cost sharing dummy variable is interpreted by Newhouse as evidence that the x-inefficiency hypothesis is valid. According to the empirical results, groups with cost sharing arrangements have average costs per visit which are $2.55 higher than those which do not. Similar regressions utilizing alternative dependent variables (e.g., medical records costs, appointment costs, and billing costs per visit) produced comparable results.

Again, however, we find that a satisfactory output measure is lacking. Newhouse has assumed away the problem of output measurement when he treats the output (an office visit) of 20 medical practices, representing eleven different medical specialties, as homogeneous. A more accurate assumption would be that outputs are different, and that the technologies used to produce them are not identical. Therefore, the test for economies of scale, or for productivity with this data, does not really have an acceptable theoretical framework. Different products cannot be compared for productivity differences, and different technologies invalidate an assumption needed to test for economies of scale.

There are a few minor problems that seem worthy of mention. Newhouse chooses to estimate an average cost curve with a U-shaped functional form. However, this seems questionable because only one of the 20 observations lies to the right of the minimum. Newhouse notes this, and suggests that the average cost curve could in fact be L-shaped, but this would then suggest constant returns to scale. Finally, his conclusion that x-inefficiency exists because of the significance of cost sharing dummy variables may also be questioned. Medical groups may have high average costs because they provide a higher quality of output or a more expensive range of services. This may be possible because they are able to share costs, whereas a solo practitioner is prohibited from providing these services. Furthermore, consideration of the revenue side, which is also shared, may also reflect the differences in the services being produced. Available data (Table 2-1) show that the average physician earns a higher income in group practice. Thus, to conclude that medical groups, by sharing costs, encourage x-inefficiency is subject to question on the basis of Newhouse's analysis. He has analyzed the cost side without considering the revenue side, and has made the questionable assumption that the outputs of these medical practices are identical. However, Newhouse's work is a major contribution to our understanding of the behavior of group practices.

Yett (1967), uses a sample from the AMA list of 1,262 self-employed physicians under age 65 to study economies of scale. He defines output as patient visits, and cost as "tax deductible professional expenses." Using a number of different cost functions, he concludes that there was evidence of economies of scale. Among other results he finds that the average expense

Table 2-1
Median Net Incomes,[a] Solo Practitioners[b] and Numbers of Partnerships,[c] 1962-1966

Year[d]	Solo Practitioners	Partners
1962	$22,800	$27,700
1963	23,300	29,150
1964	26,650	31,560
1965	26,680	33,450
1966	29,740	36,720

[a]Source: *Medical Economics*.

[b]Source: Defined as those sharing neither income nor practice expenses.

[c]Source: Reported as numbering 30 percent of all self-employed physicians under age 65.

[d]Source: The data is reported by *Medical Economics*.

function for "expense sharers" is slightly higher than for physicians who do not share, and that the average expense function for group practice was lower than for other modes of practice. Yett concludes that there was strong evidence that physician expenses are subject to economies of scale.

Again, however, the data are subject to criticism. Aside from the usual problems of cost and output measures, the study was based on only a 41 percent response rate, and only 15 percent of the sample was usable. The low R^2 (0.5), as pointed out by Yett himself, provides some evidence that the cost curve specifications used may not be correct. However, there is no rigorous way of accepting or rejecting the predetermined cost functions which were used.

There have also been other studies on economies of scale. Kovner (1968) claims that his production function for outpatient medical facilities (all members of the Southern California Kaiser Foundation Plan) demonstrates increasing returns to scale. An AMA National Survey in 1966 indicates that private physician practices had an average 2.05 visits per hour in "solo" compared to 2.18 in nonsolo practice (see Donabedian, 1969). A similar result was obtained for 1966 by *Medical Economics*, in which solo practices were found to have produced on the average 1.47 visits per hour, as compared to 1.65 in partnerships or group practices (Donabedian, 1969). However, all of the above studies suffer from deficiencies in data and measurement, and their results must be viewed with caution.

Suggested Research

On the basis of this review of the literature on the productivity of group versus solo practice, and on the related question of economies of scale, the obvious conclusion is that the research findings are mixed. As has been emphasized above, some of the differences may be attributable in part to the lack of a clear theoretical and empirical separation of the two concepts. Furthermore, comparison of these results is made more difficult because of the variety of output definitions which have been used.

One basic problem, then, is that medical practices are multiproduct firms, and the product line tends to expand as the size of the firm increases. Treating the practices as having a single production function, as all of the research to this date has, may therefore be misleading. In fact, the question of scale may be beyond the reach of existing methodology. Until dramatically improved methods can be applied then, perhaps the simpler and more methodologically consistent question of productivity difference between solo and group practice should be given priority. The current HMO proposal assumes that medical groups are more productive; thus, an empirical test of the validity of this assumption seems paramount.

Another conclusion evident throughout the paper is that the pervasive problem of output measurement remains unsolved. Kovner's use of a relative value scale is a step in the right direction, but this approach is not yet fully developed. At this time there is an acceptable output measure for single specialty clinics, but an output measure for multispecialty clinics (which have the greatest potential as HMOs) is the most difficult and least developed. Research to develop an output measure for group practice therefore warrants high priority.

No systematic study has been made of effect of prepayment on productivity. Some research (Donabedian, 1965 and 1969) suggests that Kaiser members are given treatment at a lower per unit cost, but this may be accounted for by a number of special circumstances other than the prepayment schemes—a specially selected population, and reliance on supporting facilities outside the group for expensive medical procedures, as well as for other financial support. More comprehensive study of prepayment on a large representative sample, specifically with regard to productivity, would now be in order.

Little work has been done on the effect of income sharing schemes on the productivity of the group physician. Such schemes are quite diverse, but they usually include as major elements the specialty of the physician and his years of experience. Increased shares are given by some groups for attracting and treating patients above some expected level, while other groups provide incentives for physicians to continue research and increase the status of the group. Clearly, the effect of the income sharing scheme is an important determinant of productivity, about which we know very little. Sloan's analysis, presented in the following chapter, is especially relevant here.

The manager in a medical group, and his effect on productivity, is another area for fruitful research.[18] It might be expected that as the group becomes larger, productivity would increase due to managerial efficiency. However, in most industries some output level is reached where managerial problems begin to cause diseconomies, and it is reasonable to assume that the management function is intertwined with the question of economies of scale. There appears to be almost no work in this area.[19]

Recent work by Smith, Miller, and Golladay (1972) may provide useful evidence at the microlevel. Their research helps to identify the technological processes involved in producing medical care. At this microlevel the production process can be better understood, and potential productivity gains can be more easily identified. Further work along this line would be useful.

Before large amounts of government funds are involved in Health Maintenance Organizations, a study of the productivity of multispecialty group practices would be helpful. Of all the research examined, only that by Kovner dealt with multispecialty groups, and his sample included only seven groups. A systematic study of multispecialty clinics should focus on development of an adequate output measure, on the role of the manager, on the relationship between different departments of the clinic, and on the effect of income sharing schemes on the productivity of the group. Productivity differences between prepaid and nonprepaid groups also warrant attention. Until work of the above nature is completed, however, the potential payoffs from investments in HMOs are really unknown.

Notes

1. For instance, minimizing cost for given output level, maximizing output for given costs, or maximizing profits.

2. The discussion above assumes that all factors increase proportionately so that any increase in output is due entirely to a change of scale. A "returns to scale" or "economies of scale" parameter can still be estimated from actual data even as scale and factor proportions vary.

3. Reder (1969) proposes to measure quality changes by (1) age-sex specific mortality rates, (2) rates of undetected illness and (3) rates of improper treatment of specific ailments.

4. As far as the author is aware, this method has not been successfully implemented.

5. See Newhouse (1973).

6. He suggests the use of periodic surveys of physician use by individuals to determine the productivity of fee for service medical care.

7. The use of casemix as an output measure has been investigated in hospitals; see Rafferty (1971) and Feldstein (1968).

8. For an excellent discussion of the point, see Auster, Leveson, and Sarachek (1969) and Grossman (1972).

9. Details on Bailey's empirical work will be discussed in the section on economies of scale.

10. Again the reader is referred to the section on economies of scale for Bailey's empirical work.

11. This criticism has been pointed out by Reder (1969).

12. There is no evidence to my knowledge to support the assumption.

13. It should be noted that Reinhardt (1970) did work with other functions as well.

14. Recall that productivity and economies of scale were both defined in terms of points on the production function.

15. Furthermore, even the variation which did exist was very small.

16. The sample consists of eleven solo, five two-man, one three-man, and two five-man practices.

17. Obviously, only medical groups share costs.

18. Note that it is methodologically consistent to treat the addition of a manager as a change in the production function of the group.

19. In an unpublished paper, Egan (1969) made some attempt to account for the management function but the question of scale was not examined directly.

Bibliography

Auster, Richard; Irving Leveson; and Deborah Sarachek, "The Production of Health, an Explanatory Study," *Journal of Human Resources*, Vol. 4, No. 4: 411-36 (February 1969).

Bailey, R.M., "A Comparison of Internists in Solo and Fee-for-Service Group Practice in the San Francisco Bay Area," *Bulletin of the New York Academy of Medicine*, Vol. 44: 1293-1303 (November 1968).

———, "Economies of Scale in Medical Practice," in *Empirical Studies in Health Economies*, edited by Herbert E. Klarman. Baltimore: The Johns Hopkins Press, 1970.

Donabedian, A., "An Evaluation of Prepaid Group Practice," *Inquiry*, Vol. 6, No. 3: 3-27 (September 1969).

———, *A Review of Some Experiences with Prepaid Group Practice*. Ann Arbor: School of Public Health, University of Michigan, 1965.

Egan, D.M., "Income and Productivity of Physicians in Fee-for-Service, Multi-Specialty Group Practice," paper prepared for the Western Economic Association Meetings, Long Beach, California, August 1969 (mimeographed).

Feldstein, M., *Economic Analysis for Health Service Efficiency Econometric Studies of the British National Health Service*. Chicago: Markham Publishing Company, 1968.

Graham, F.E., "Group Versus Solo Practice: Arguments and Evidence," *Inquiry*, Vol. 9, No. 2: 49-60, (June 1972).

Grossman, Michael, "On the Concept of Health Capital and the Demand for Health," *Journal of Political Economy*, Vol. 80, No. 2: 223-55 (April 1972).

Kovner, J.W., "A Production Function for Outpatient Medical Facilities," unpublished Ph.D. dissertation, University of California, Los Angeles, 1968.

Newhouse, J.P., "The Economics of Group Practice," *Journal of Human Resources*, Vol. 8, No. 1: 174-83, (Winter 1973).

Olson, M., *The Logic of Collective Action*. Cambridge, Mass.: Harvard University Press, 1965.

Rafferty, John A., "Patterns of Hospital Use: An Analysis of Short-Run Variation," *Journal of Political Economy*, Vol. 79, No. 1: 154-65, (January/February 1971).

Reder, M.W., "Some Problems in the Measurement of Productivity in the Medical Care Industry," in *Production and Productivity in the Service Industries*, edited by Victor R. Fuchs. New York: Columbia University Press, 1969.

Reinhardt, U.E., "An Economic Analysis of Physicians' Practices," unpublished Ph.D. dissertation, Yale University, 1970.

———, "A Production Function for Physicians' Services," *Review of Economics and Statistics* (February 1972).

Scheffler, R.M., "Estimated Rate of Return to the Physician's Assistant," *Industrial Relations* (forthcoming 1974).

_____ , "Further Consideration in the Economics of Group Practice: The Management Input," Working paper, The University of North Carolina, Chapel Hill (1974).

_____ , "The Pricing Behavior of Medical Groups," Working paper, The University of North Carolina, Chapel Hill (1974).

_____ , "The Market for Paraprofessionals: The Physician Assistant," *The Quarterly Review of Economics and Business* (forthcoming, Fall, 1974).

Smith, K.R.; Marriane Miller, and Frederick L. Golladay, "An Analysis of the Optimal Use of Inputs in the Production of Medical Services," *Journal of Human Resources*, Vol. 2: 208-25 (Spring 1972).

U.S. Department of Health, Education, and Welfare, "Studies of the Incomes of Physicians and Dentists," by Louis S. Reed, Social Security Administration, Office of Research and Statistics, December 1968.

U.S. Department of Health, Education, and Welfare, "Towards a Comprehensive Health Policy for the 1970—A White Paper," May 1971.

Yankauer, A., J.P. Connelly; and J.J. Feldman, "Physician Productivity in the Delivery of Ambulatory Care: Some Findings from a Survey of Pediatricians," *Medical Care*, Vol.8, No. 1: 35-46 (January/February 1970).

Yett, D.E., "An Evaluation of Alternative Methods of Estimating Physician's Expenses Relative to Output," *Inquiry*, Vol. 4: 3-27 (March 1967).

Effects of Incentives on Physician Performance

Frank A. Sloan*

Introduction

Recent increases in demand for medical services, in large part a response to a rapidly expanding federal role, have led to numerous policy statements concerning an apparent shortage of medical personnel. Much policymaker interest has focused on the physician. Recommended methods for augmenting the effective supply, both in the short- and long-run, abound. One of the short or immediate run "solutions" is to increase physician productivity by encouraging group practices.[1] However, whether or not encouraging physicians to join groups is a desirable policy remains to be demonstrated.

The relative merits of alternative modes of practice may be expressed in terms of both efficiency and effectiveness. Aspects of allocative and scale efficiency have already been discussed in this volume. Technical or x-efficiency has not.[2] But if decision making within groups primarily takes place at the individual group member level, then practice output, price, and input purchase decisions will reflect individual member marginal costs and returns rather than those of the group. Although the individual physician in the group would earn more if these choices were centralized, he may be willing to forego income to maintain a degree of independence. However, the principal reason for policy concern is not the potential physician income loss, but rather that incentives inherent in groups may reduce productivity; they may result in lower output, at a higher resource cost per unit.

The major objective of this chapter is to suggest fruitful directions for future research on this important issue. The following section first develops physician decision-making models in the context of cost-sharing and revenue-cost sharing practice. It recasts a hypothesis stated in Newhouse (1973) in somewhat more formal terms.[3] Total scale-adjusted, nonphysician costs rise as the group size increases because the individual physician member bears an increasingly smaller proportion of the financial consequences of his failure to control costs. Where both revenues and costs are shared, the financial return to individual effort falls as group size rises. A negative relationship between effort and group size is

*Associate Professor of Economics and Community Health and Family Medicine, University of Florida. The author wishes to thank Roger Blair, Joseph Newhouse, and Bruce Steinwald for helpful comments on an earlier draft.

predicted when both revenues and costs are shared. We then discuss the implications of these physician decision-making models, and present institutional evidence on group management structure and revenue-cost sharing arrangements. Although information is fragmentary, there is some evidence that management becomes more centralized as the number of physicians in the group rises. The empirical evidence does not refute the conceptual models, but this evidence does suggest that there have been some institutional responses to counterpotential disincentives. Therefore, previously published evidence is reviewed on comparative physician costs, output, and effort (as measured by the length of the work week and the number of weeks worked per year) by practice type and size.

Research on physician choice of practice mode and the effects of incentives inherent in alternative modes are closely related. If there are systematic preference differences among physicians selecting various modes, estimates of the effect of incentives on practice efficiency may be biased. Thus, we review recent surveys on factors affecting practice mode choice, and present the available evidence. The last portion of the chapter summarizes the study and suggests future research directions.

Models

This section develops models reflecting differences in incentives inherent in alternative organizational forms of physician practice. Given these structural differences, the models are used to predict the effect of incentives on practice output, price, and input purchase decisions. The vast majority of patient-care physicians practice under fee-for-service reimbursement arrangements. The emphasis in this section, therefore, is on fee-for-service. However, as seen toward the end of the section, the methodology is readily transferrable to salary and capitation arrangements financed on a prepaid basis.

Fee-for-service physicians may share costs and revenue under numerous types of arrangements. Cost-sharing may include fixed and/or variable costs. In the context of medical practice, examples of fixed costs are capital equipment items, such as an X-ray unit or a building, or personnel embodying a substantial amount of practice-specific training. Variable costs are supplies, purchased laboratory services, and some labor with comparatively little specific training. Under revenue-cost (or income) sharing arrangements, net income may be divided among group members in equal or unequal shares.

The following models of physician decision making assume that physicians behave as profit maximizers in decisions affecting output, price, and input costs and that each physician member of a group exercises a substantial degree of individual discretion in making these decisions. The models incorporate a term to represent the value the physician imputes to his foregone leisure. Thus, profits represent the difference between total revenue and a total cost that includes the physician's imputed wage. The assumption that price, output, and input decisions are guided by profit maximization does not preclude nonpecuniary factors from affecting other types of decisions, e.g., specialty choice or, for that matter, choice of practice mode (determined prior to the output, price, and input decisions).

This section investigates the effects of individual decision making within a group context. Whether or not, and under what circumstances, this assumption is reasonable will subsequently be investigated.

Cost-Sharing

Assume that the physician's cost function is

$$C = c_0 + (c_1 + c_2)q + (c_3/n) + (c_4/n)q. \tag{3.1}$$

According to (3.1), he pays all of certain fixed costs (c_0), certain marginal costs (c_1), but shares other fixed (c_3) and marginal (c_4) costs; n denotes the size of the cost-sharing group. c_2 is the imputed marginal cost per visit (q), the product of the value of a minute of foregone leisure and the mean length of a visit. Assume that c_2 is constant. (It may be easily shown that allowing marginal cost to vary positively with output yields the same (qualitative) predictions.) In addition, assume that the physician's demand curve is given by

$$p = a_0 + a_1q + a_2Z \tag{3.2}$$

where p is the price of a visit, and Z, any other factor affecting demand. Each physician in the cost-sharing group sets his own price. Furthermore, assume (as is reasonable) no price competition among group members. Then, the individual physician's net income or profit (Y) (taking the imputed value of his leisure into account) is

$$Y = (a_0 + a_1q + a_2Z)q - [c_0 + (c_1 + c_2)q + (c_3/n) + (c_4/n)q]. \tag{3.3}$$

Equation (3.3) may be appropriate, for example, if the physician practices in two locations; he shares total costs in one but not the other location. If all costs are shared, c_0 and c_1 are zero. c_2 is nevertheless positive. Differentiating (3.3) with respect to q, q^*, the optimal number of visits supplied is

$$q^* = (1/2a_1) [-a_0 - a_2Z + (c_1 + c_2) + (c_4/n)]. \tag{3.4}$$

Corresponding to q^* is the physician's price per visit

$$p^* = (1/2) [a_0 + a_2Z + (c_1 + c_2) + (c_4/n)]. \tag{3.5}$$

According to (3.4) and (3.5), quantity is higher and price lower, the larger the size of the group, holding c_1 and c_2 constant. Assuming c_3 and c_4 are independent of n, the incentive to reduce shared costs varies inversely with n. This is seen by substituting (3.4) and (3.5) into (3.3) and total differentiating. Setting all differentials but those pertaining to shared costs equal to zero, the total derivative of Y reduces to

$$dY = -(1/n)dc_3 - (1/2a_1 n)[-a_0 - a_2 Z + (c_1 + c_2) + (c_4/n)]dc_4. \quad (3.6)$$

From (3.6), $dY/dc_3 = (1/n)$. That is, a dollar reduction in shared fixed costs increases the physician's income (adjusted for foregone leisure) by an amount proportionate to the reciprocal of the number of fixed cost sharers. Since *both* the expression in brackets and a_1 are negative, dY/dc_4 is negative.[4] The gain from a dollar decrease in the shared marginal cost depends in part on the a's, Z, c_1, and c_2, but the gain is smaller when n is large. But if the rise in cost stemming from a decreased incentive to the individual physician to be efficient in his practice is sufficiently great, the conclusions based on Equations (3.4) and (3.5) need not hold. The derivative, $dq*/dn = (1/2a_1)(-c_4/n^2)$, is positive if c_4 is independent of n. But if c_4 varies directly with n, then it is easily shown that $dq*/dn$ is only positive only if $|c_4/n|$, the individual physician's share of shared marginal costs, exceeds $|dc_4/dn|$, the change in efficiency consciousness as practice size increases.

The marginal income gain to the individual physician from increasing the size of the cost-sharing group, holding scale effects constant, may be derived from the total differential of Y, with all differentials except dn equal to zero.[5]

$$dY/dn = (c_3/n^2) + (c_4/2a_1 n^2)[-a_0 - a_2 Z + (c_1 + c_2) + (c_4/n)]. \quad (3.7)$$

As in Equation (3.6), the expression in brackets is negative, and dY/dn is thus positive. Using the above cost function and assuming costs are distributed independently of n, members gain by adding physicians to the cost-sharing group, and the incentive to do so is greater if the shared costs are high. However, the derivative of dY/dn is negative, indicating that dY/dn declines as group size increases. If c_3 and c_4 are positive functions of n, then a term

$$- (dc_3/dn)(1/n) - (1/2a_1)(dc_1/dn)(1/n)$$

$$[-a_0 - a_2 Z + (c_1 + c_2) + c_4(n)/n]$$

which is negative, must be added to (3.7). The derivative dY/dn may be negative for certain nonzero values of dc_3/dn and dc_1/dn. If dc_3/dn and dc_1/dn are small, but negative, one should observe groups of all sizes being formed.

The above discussion leads one to predict that quantity will rise and price fall, *ceteris paribus*, as n increases if n does *not* affect the shared marginal cost c_4. Likewise, the gain to the individual physician from reductions in shared costs varies negatively with the size of the group. Finally, there are private monetary returns from cost-sharing, but these depend on the amount of costs to be shared and the marginal return from increasing n diminishes as n grows large. Although these results follow rather easily from standard assumptions, they also provide an indication of problems in empirical research on the topic. Physicians with high fixed and marginal costs have more to gain from sharing, but once in a group, sharers experience a lower return from cost-cutting than nonsharers. A more realistic specification may be to make c_3 and c_4 functions of n. If dc_3/dn and dc_4/dn are high and positive, the conclusions are reversed. Output falls as does the individual physician's financial incentive to form cost-sharing groups.[6]

Revenue-Cost Sharing: Equal Shares

To analyze the effects of income sharing on both costs and productivity, respecify (3.1) as

$$C = c_0 + c_1 q + (n-1)\,\overline{C}(\overline{q}) + c_2 q. \tag{3.8}$$

$C(q)$ denotes total costs, excluding imputed time costs, of each of the other physician members of the group, which by assumption are exogenous to individual members. The demand function for other members is

$$(n-1)\overline{p} = (n-1)\overline{a}_0 + (n-1)\overline{a}_1\overline{q} + (n-1)\overline{a}_2\overline{Z}; \tag{3.9}$$

total group profits (with revenues and costs of one "representative" member expressed separately) are

$$\pi = (a_0 + a_1 q + a_2 Z)q - c_0 - c_1 q + (n-1) \tag{3.10}$$
$$[\overline{a}_0 + \overline{a}_1\overline{q} + \overline{a}_2\overline{Z}]\,\overline{q} - (n-1)\overline{C}(\overline{q}).$$

Assuming that the individual member treats the decisions of the others as fixed and income of the group is shared equally among the members,

$$Y = (1/n)\big\{(a_0 + a_1 q + a_2 Z)q - c_0 - c_1 q + (n-1) \tag{3.11}$$
$$[(a_0 + a_1 q + a_2 Z)q - C(q)]\big\} - c_2 q.$$

Although the members may share all nonphysician practice costs, it is not feasible to share the physician's personal costs which depend on his effort. Differentiating Y with respect to q,

$$q* - (1/2a_1) [-a_0 Z + c_1 + nc_2].$$ (3.12)

If the implicit personal cost (c_2) were zero, income-sharing would have no impact on the optimal quantity supplied. But according to (3.12), as n increases, $q*$ decreases (again, since a_1 is negative). In contrast to cost-sharing, $q*$ is lower for income-sharing physicians, even if the c's do not depend on n. Substituting $q*$ into the demand relationship,

$$p* = 1/2 [a_0 + a_2 Z + c_1 + nc_2].$$ (3.13)

As n increases, so does price.

All fee-for-service derivations in this section are based on the assumption of price-setting by individual members. This assumption may be more appropriate for multispecialty than for single-specialty and general practice groups. In the former, the services offered by each member may be relatively unique. However, even if prices are exogenous to individual members, this does not alter the basic conclusions with respect to individual output decisions and individual motivations to reduce costs. Although empirical evidence is lacking, it is probably true that customary fees for a specific procedure are reasonably uniform within a group. But this does not mean that price decisions are primarily the result of group rather than individual decision making. A physician who performs the procedure frequently may be the effective price-setter. Moreover, once the customary fee has been set, individual members undoubtedly exercise considerable discretion in determining the average price of the procedure. For example, the member may determine in a specific instance whether or not the full, customary fee will be charged to a patient.[7]

Substituting (3.12) and (3.13) into (3.11), individual physician income is

$$Y = (1/n) \big\{ (1/4a_1) [-a_0 - a_2 Z + c_1 + nc_2] \cdot$$ (3.14)

$$[-a_0 - a_2 Z + c_1 + nc_2] - c_0 - c_1 \cdot$$

$$(1/2a_1) [-a_0 - a_2 Z + c_1 + nc_2] + (n - 1)$$

$$[(\overline{a}_0 + \overline{a}_1 \overline{q} + \overline{a}_2 Z)\overline{q}] - (n - 1) \overline{C}(\overline{q}) \big\} - c_2 (1/2a_1) \cdot$$

$$[-a_0 - a_2 Z + c_1 + nc_2] \cdot$$

$$dY/dc_0 = -(1/n) \text{ and } dY/dc_1 = -(1/2a_1 n) [-a_0 - a_2 Z + c_1 + nc_2].$$

Both derivatives are negative. For high c_2, the incentive to the individual physician member of an equal income-sharing group to reduce nonphysician marginal costs (c_1) is relatively low.

Letting Y_m be income exclusive of the $c_2 (1/2a_1) [-a_0 - a_2 Z + c_1 + nc_2]$

component of (3.14), one may then calculate the earnings loss (as opposed to the loss that takes the value of foregone leisure into account) from an increase in the imputed cost per visit c_2. $dY_m/dc_2 = nc_2/a_1$. This derivative is negative and becomes more so when a_1 is low; then, the number of visits demanded is relatively responsive to price, and the income loss from a rise in price is correspondingly large. The derivative dY_m/dc_2 also depends on n; when n is large, dY_m/dc_2 declines more because the individual's output restriction in response to a rise in c_2 is greater under these circumstances.[8]

Equation (3.11) is sufficiently general to permit analysis of physicians with unequal demand and cost structures (since an "a" or "c" of the "representative" physician need not equal its counterpart, "$\overline{a}$" or "$\overline{c}$"). Let $p = l(a_0 + a_1 q + n_2 Z)$, where l is a demand shift factor for the individual physician, then it is easily seen that individual physician output increases if l exceeds one. But the disincentive effect of group size remains the same. Physicians who consistently contribute a relatively large portion of total income to an equal income-sharing group have a financial incentive to leave the organization.

Revenue-Cost Sharing: Unequal Shares

Equation (3.11) may be modified for analysis of groups sharing net income on an unequal shares basis. One basis for unequal sharing may be on the basis of seniority and/or the individual member's investment in the group practice. Then, θ_i, the share of the ith member, is substituted for $1/n$ in (3.11).

$$Y = \theta_i \left\{ (a_0 + a_1 q + a_2 Z)q - c_0 - c_1 q(n-1) \cdot \right. \tag{3.11$'$}$$

$$\left. [(\overline{a}_0 + \overline{a}_1 \overline{q} + \overline{a}_2 \overline{Z})\overline{q}] - (n-1)\overline{C}(\overline{q}) \right\} - c_2 q$$

$$\sum_{i=1}^{n} \theta_i = 1.$$

Quantity, price, and input purchase decisions now depend on θ_i. As θ_i becomes large, output supplied by the individual member increases, price falls, and the individual incentives to reduce shared costs rise. It follows directly from derivatives of (3.11$'$) that if c_2 varies directly with physician age, and if θ_i rises with seniority, a rising θ_i will provide an offset to a rising c_2.[9] In reality, it may often be difficult to assess the wage individual members of a group impute to their foregone leisure.

Another form of unequal income-sharing is to allow the physician to retain a fraction of group profits directly attributable to him (Y_i), a share that is larger than $1/n$, and in addition make a flat payment to him from the profits remaining. Then Equation (3.11) becomes

$$Y = \gamma_i [(a_0 + a_1 q + a_2 Z)q - c_0 - c_1 q] + \left\{ [(n - \sum_{i=1}^{n} \gamma_i)(n-1)] / n \right\} \cdot$$

$$[(\overline{a}_0 + \overline{a}_1 \overline{q} + \overline{a}_2 \overline{Z})\overline{q} - \overline{C}(\overline{q})] - c_2 q. \tag{3.11''}$$

In contrast to (3.11'), which involves raising output and cost reduction incentives for some, but reducing them for others, (3.11'') raises individual incentives for all (and at the same time increases the variance in income to individual members). In the limit ($\gamma_i = 1$ for all members), there is no income-sharing at all. For any γ_i less than one, income-sharing will produce disincentive effects.

There are still other methods for distributing practice income among members on an unequal basis, but these are less tractable analytically. If θ_i or γ_i depends on the member's fraction of visits of total visits for the group, or alternatively, on the member's fraction of total group billings, third degree terms appear in the first order conditions, even if linear cost and demand functions are employed. But sharing on a visits basis is only likely in single-specialty practice since there are considerable interspecialty differences in the medical resource commitment per visit. If individual physician billings provide the basis for allocating gross revenue, but *not* costs, this type of arrangement is a cost-sharing scheme and may be analyzed according to methods given above. Or if the fraction depends on past revenue performance and the individual member is quite uncertain about current output-price decisions of others in the group, the fraction may be regarded as fixed, and analysis of the billings-based arrangements follows from either (3.11') or (3.11''). Only if the sharing proportions and output-price decisions are determined simultaneously and both revenues and costs are shared on the basis of member billings does an analytical problem exist. Available descriptions on billings-oriented sharing schemes are often too vague to distinguish among these variants.

Nonfee-for-Service Practices

If physicians compensated on a salaried basis derive no nonpecuniary benefits from providing additional units of patient care, it follows from the above framework that they will produce at the minimum acceptable level. If salary is a function of past effort, they *may* work above the minimum.[10]

Under capitation arrangements, physicians are compensated on the basis of the number of patient enrollees or subscribers. If the group must provide a minimum level of service to have any subscribers at all, and providing additional patient benefits beyond this level has no impact on the number of subscribers, performance under capitation arrangements should be identical to salaried practice.[11] But, if the group providing more services per subscriber obtains more subscribers, there are important differences.

Let $S = b_0 + b_1 q + b_2 (n - 1)\overline{q}$, $\qquad\qquad$ (3.15)

where S is the number of subscribers to the plan. Let

$$r = d_0 + d_1 S + d_2 W, \qquad\qquad (3.16)$$

where r is the capitation rate per subscriber and W, exogenous factors affecting demand. Then assuming equal income-sharing, income for each individual member is given by

$$Y = (1/n) [rS - c_0 - c_1 q - (n - 1)\overline{C}(\overline{q})] - c_2 q. \qquad (3.17)$$

Substituting (3.15) and (3.16) into (3.17),

$$Y = (1/n) \left\{ [d_0 + d_1 (b_0 + b_1 q + b_2 (n - 1)\overline{q}) + d_2 W] \cdot \right. \qquad (3.18)$$
$$\left. [b_0 + b_1 q + b_2 (n - 1)\overline{q}] - c_0 - c_1 q - (n - 1)\overline{C}(\overline{q}) \right\} - c_2 q'$$

Differentiating (3.18), and solving for $q*$,

$$q* = (1/2b_1 d_1)[-d_2 W + (c_1 + nc_2)/b_1] - \qquad (3.19)$$
$$(1/b_1) [b_0 + d_0/2 + b_2 (n - 1)\overline{q}].$$

As before, the individual member's output decreases as n grows large. An essential difference is that under capitation (according to the above specification), output of other members affects individual decisions. $dq*/dq = b_2$ $(n-1)/b_1$, which is negative. If the individual member anticipates that his partners will be industrious, his output diminishes, and the reverse holds if his partners are not expected to be diligent. This factor tends to stabilize output of the group. Because patient demand under capitation is much more likely to be directed toward the physician group as a whole rather than toward its individual members, as in fee-for-service practice, $\overline{q}$ is more likely to enter the individual physician member's output decision under capitation.

Hypotheses

The theoretical section provides the basis for several hypotheses concerning incentives affecting practice costs and productivity in various settings. Cost-sharing physicians should set quantity higher and price lower than their non-cost-sharing colleagues. However, the incentive to reduce costs is lower under cost-sharing and this incentive diminishes as the size of the group increases. If the cost parameters vary directly with group size, which is plausible, quantity is lower and price higher.

Income (or revenue-cost) sharing groups may take several forms. Apportioning net practice income for the group among physicians equally, the model predicts that output will be lower for higher group size; it will also be lower if the cost imputed to foregone leisure by the physician is higher. Price varies directly with both group size and the imputed costs. As in cost-sharing practice, the income gain to the individual physician from a reduction in either fixed and/or marginal costs is inversely proportional to group size. Unequal demand for individual members within the equal sharing group does not alter these conclusions, but equal sharing will not be attractive to the physician with high relative demand and/or low costs.

Numerous types of unequal income-sharing schemes exist. Individual members may receive unequal shares of the total net income of the group, or greater weight (than $1/n$) may be given to revenues and costs attributed to each individual member with a corresponding lower weight on the net income generated by other group members. The former method mitigates the disincentive effects of large group size for members receiving more than $1/n$ of group net revenue, but increases it for those who receive a smaller proportion than $1/n$. Weighing the individual contribution more heavily raises quantity and lowers price, and raises physician cost-consciousness.

Using Section I-type models, salaried practice appears very unattractive in terms of physician effort. Workloads would be expected to fall to a minimum "acceptable" level. Moreover, there is no incentive under this arrangement for individual physicians to monitor costs. Capitation practices are distinguished by having a group demand schedule rather than schedules for individual members. These ways of specifying demand are not fully appropriate for either practice arrangement, but there is a tendency for demand under capitation to be more oriented toward the group than is the case under fee-for-service practice. The major consequence of group demand is that individual member output depends (negatively) on the output of other members. This factor would tend to equalize effort among members. However, disincentive effects associated with size remain.

The above predictions follow directly from the assumptions. In general, large size is associated with reduced incentives for the individual physician. Whether or not groups realize this problem and have modified the incentive structures of their practices to mitigate the effects of size is a question to be decided on the basis of empirical evidence.

Empirical Evidence: Group Management
and Cost-Sharing

Unfortunately, model-building and data collection often proceed independently, and surveys of group practice have generally been no exception. To truly understand the incentive structures inherent in alternative practice forms, it is important to identify the locus of decision making within the group. If some decisions are made jointly and others individually, it is useful to know which decision is made at what level.

Surveys have been based on essentially two concepts of groups. Some well-known surveys prior to 1960, most notable Rorem (1931), Hunt and Goldstein (1951), and the 1959 Public Health Service study [(United States Public Health Service 1963)], make income-pooling a prerequisite for including a practice in their surveys. More recent surveys by the American Medical Association [Balfe and McNamara (1968) and Todd and McNamara (1971)] only require that the members distribute income according to a "prearranged plan." Thus, the more recent surveys are more likely to include cost-sharing groups than are several earlier ones. Nevertheless, some cost-sharing physician respondents to the American Medical Association surveys may have taken the definition to imply income-pooling and, as a result, failed to respond to the questionnaire. The evidence from the surveys is probably much more closely related to income than to cost-sharing groups.[12]

That individual members in groups have less incentive to control costs than do solo practitioners and that this incentive varies inversely with group size are important predictions of the above models. Yet, if there is a method for representing the collective interests of the individual members, the relative lack of cost-consciousness as n grows large need never occur. Indeed, as Table 3-1 indicates, the propensity of groups to organize a board of directors and/or a group manager increases with group size. Either a board or a manager can screen requests for additional personnel and equipment to insure that these requests are consistent with maximum profits for the group as a whole. Whether or not the managerial structure performs this function adequately is an empirical issue worthy of further study. The data suggests, nevertheless, that physicians in groups are aware of the consequence of individual actions, at least to a limited extent, and that mechanisms with the potential of collectivizing the decision making process have been established. According to Table 3-1, physicians in multispecialty groups are more likely to have a formal managerial structure than those in single specialty or general practice groups. Multispecialty groups are larger, and this pattern could reflect relative size. However, it is also possible that the opportunities for expenditures (from the group's vantage point) are greater in this type of group because physicians in one specialty may be rather poor judges of whether expenditures related to another field will increase group profits. A formal review mechanism may compensate for this lack of knowledge on the part of individual members.

Research on the managerial structure of groups is clearly needed. A factor that should be included in the analysis is the method for compensating the manager. If he is partially compensated under a profit-sharing scheme, one would expect him to be more sensitive to practice purchase decisions. There is

Table 3-1
Group Management

A. *Number of Groups with to Those Without a Board of Directors*

					Size of Group					
	3	*4*	*5*	*6*	*7*	*8-15*	*16-25*	*26-49*	*50-99*	*100+*	*All*
Ratio	0.45	0.75	1.13	1.64	1.67	2.99	9.27	18.20	32.00	[a]	0.87

	Type of Group		
	Single Specialty	*General Practice*	*Multispecialty*
Ratio	0.65	0.56	1.44

B. *Number of Groups with to Those Without a Board of Directors*

					Size of Group					
	3	*4*	*5*	*6*	*7*	*8-15*	*16-25*	*26-59*	*50-99*	*100+*	*All*
Ratio	0.22	0.37	0.60	0.84	0.93	2.38	14.30	31.30	15.50	16.00	0.51

	Type of Group		
	Single Specialty	*General Practice*	*Multispecialty*
Ratio	0.25	0.39	1.16

Source: Todd and McNamara (1971). Data pertain to 1969. "a" indicates all groups in the cell have a board of directors.

probably less that a manager is able to accomplish on the revenue than on the cost side to increase group profits.

Both physician production per hour and the number of hours he works should partially reflect the method used to distribute practice profits among individual physician members. Table 3-2 shows methods of income distribution by types of group. Salary or salary plus a share of net income are not prevalent physician compensation arrangements in any of the three group types. Most groups compensate on the basis of a share of net income. As one would expect, single specialty and general practice groups divide net income of the group equally more often than do multispecialty groups. This result is not surprising if only because there is considerable interspecialty variation in income per hour of work. Physicians in high net revenue fields would be expected to be less willing to join groups on an equal share basis. A more interesting result, seen from Table 3-3, is that varying share arrangements become common as group size increases, holding group type constant. However, this pattern is not as distinct as that between management structure and group size. The few cases where varying

Table 3-2
Groups by Method of Income Distribution

Method of Income Distribution	Total	Type of Group		
		Single Specialty	General Practice	Multispecialty
Salary only	156 (3.6)	6464 (3.0)	12 (1.8)	80 (5.4)
Salary plus a share of net income	168 (3.9)	69 (3.2)	12 (1.8)	87 (5.9)
Share of net income:				
equal share	1,587 (37.0)	919 (42.6)	300 (46.1)	368 (24.9)
varying share	1,976 (46.1)	919 (42.6)	263 (40.4)	794 (53.8)
Other and no answer	402 (9.4)	190 (8.8)	64 (9.8)	148 (10.0)
Total	4,289 (100.0)	2,161 (100.0)	651 (100.0)	1,477 (100.0)

Source: Balfe and McNamara (1968). Data pertains to 1965.

shares do not increase with group size probably reflect sample variability in part. Stratifying by both group type and size results in a few small cells.

There are several types of arrangements under the category "varying share of net income." According to Balfe and McNamara (1968), the term includes a wide variety of income distribution arrangements. Of the 1,976 groups in this category, 26.1 percent divided income among members according to the number of individual bookings (dollar amount of fees charged) accountable to each physician.[13] The remaining 73.9 percent allocated income according to some formula determined by the group members. Among these were 319 who stated explicitly that they use the point system, a general term for several systems which assign points to individual physicians according to some predetermined criteria. Rorem (1931) and the United States Public Health Service (1963) give several examples of income-sharing schemes. Even though this information

Table 3-3
Method of Income Distribution: Ratio to Equal Income Sharers to Varying Income Sharers by Size and Type of Group

Type of Group	Size of Group								
	3	4	5	6	7	8-15	16-25	26-49	All
Single specialty	1.08	0.94	0.87	0.89	1.59	0.86	a	a	1.00
General practice	1.34	0.82	0.72	a	a	a	a	a	1.14
Multispecialty	0.52	0.67	0.51	0.41	0.64	0.33	0.31	0.26	0.46

Source: Balfe and McNamara (1968). "a" indicates there are fewer than 10 observations in the cell.

cannot be used for determining relative frequencies of various methods of sharing, seniority and/or sharing based on investments in the group appear in a large proportion of the examples they present.

Although it appears that groups often attempt to counterbalance the disincentive effects of size by instituting varying shares, more detailed data would be useful. The reward from additional effort is less to physicians in groups which distribute income on a equal share than on an unequal basis, and the difference is even more pronounced if one compares unequal income with salaried practice. But there is undoubtedly considerable variation in incentives at the margin within the "varying share" category which cannot be determined with available evidence.

Empirical Evidence: Cost and Productivity in Alternative Practice Setting

Methodological Problems

Cost and productivity data by practice type is available from several published sources. In general, this data is presented in tabular form; thus multivariate analysis, which has the potential of isolating the independent effect of the incentive structure, cannot be performed with this data. Even if large quantities of raw data were available and the incentive structure could be measured with greater precision than has been accomplished to date, empirical research relating incentive structure to practice costs and productivity would likely encounter several methodological difficulties. The most important are these:

First, physicians who anticipate high practice costs (for example, for malpractice insurance or expensive laboratory equipment) are more likely to desire to pool expenses with others than those with lower cost expectations. In the context of insurance, this is termed the "adverse selection problem." It is appropriate to attribute high relative costs to the incentive structure if they reflect a lack of incentive to be cost-conscious. However, identifying the response to incentives may be difficult if causality also runs from expected cost to the incentive.

Second, if one is to attribute relatively low levels of physician effort to group size, n must vary independently of c_2, the physician's imputed cost. But, the two may be positively associated. That is, physicians who place a relatively high value on leisure may choose practice settings in which there is comparatively little pressure on them to treat many patients per hour or work many hours. If so, what appears to be a "group size" effect on physician output is, at least in part, a "taste" effect. More must be known about the preferences of physicians choosing alternative practice structures. Responses to incentive should not be studied in isolation.

Three, case-mix differences may account for some of the apparent variation in cost and productivity. Specifically, large clinics treat more difficult cases, often referred from smaller, less specialized practices. This reason for apparent relative inefficiency is often cited by professionals associated with large clinics. Although this may be an excuse which is used to obscure apparent inefficiency, there is undoubtedly some merit to their argument as well.

Because of these potential methodological difficulties and the aggregate nature of available data, the following evidence on cost and productivity performance in alternative practice settings should be considered tentative.

Costs

Taylor and Newhouse (1970) and Newhouse (1973) report overhead costs per patient visit (all nonphysician costs except costs of ancillary services and space) to be far greater in three outpatient clinics ($14.24) than in a small sample of private practice physicians they surveyed ($4.54). Both solo and group practices are included in the private practice sample; the largest of these is considerably smaller (measured in terms of the number of patient visits) than the smallest of the three outpatient clinics. Sloan (1971) reports the average labor cost per visit (including the physician) of three community mental health center outpatient clinics to be $21.93, $52.13, and $27.16 for late 1969 and early 1970. By comparison, the mean charges on a national basis for first and follow-up office visits according to the American Medical Association were $32.64 and $29.50, respectively. The national mean charges presumably cover physician time, other labor, as well as capital costs. Moreover, they refer to individual patient contacts with a psychiatrist. By contrast, more therapist contacts in the three clinics were to groups of patients; each patient contact counted as a visit. Unlike private practice, the therapist in the clinic was often a nonpsychiatrist. Both studies report a substantial amount of time spent by staff to non-patient-related functions. This data suggests a lack of incentive for efficient production within institutional (salaried) practice.

Table 3-4 gives data on practice expenses (excluding the physician) per visit for 1969-1970. This data is even lower than the Taylor-Newhouse private practice estimates, in part reflecting definitional differences and because Taylor-Newhouse's data pertains to a major metropolitan area rather than to the nation as a whole. According to Table 3-4, groups, primarily fee-for-service, have the lowest expense-visit ratio. This data suggests that something other than size per se can explain the differences between outpatient clinic and private practice expenses. Of course, the comparisons would be more definitive if the group category were disaggregated by size of practice.

Table 3-4
Weeks Worked, Visits, and Expenses per Visit

A. Physicians in All Fields[a]

Type of Patients	Weeks Worked	Direct Hours Worked	Total Hours Worked	Visits	Expense/ Visits
Solo	48.1	45.6	50.9	126.5 (2.77)	$3.75
Two-man partnership	48.2	47.9	53.9	158.2 (30)	3.56
Informal association	48.3	49.1	55.3	132.2 (2.69)	3.71
Group	47.8	47.0	53.5	156.4 (3.33)	2.97

Major Source of Income

Fee-for-services only	–	47.1	52.3	141.8 (3.0)	–
Fee-for-service with some salary	–	43.7	51.4	123.0 (2.8)	–
Salary with some fee-for-service	–	35.3	48.3	98.1 (2.8)	–
Salary only	–	34.9	46.6	102.7 (2.9)	–
Retainer only	–	43.0	44.0	102.8 (2.4)	–

B. Internists[b]

Type of Practice

Solo	–	48.4	–	– (3.4)	–
Two-man partnership	–	49.3	–	– (3.0)	–
Three-man group	–	43.8	–	– (3.5)	–
Four-to-five man group	–	44.4	–	– (3.1)	–
Clinics	–	43.8	–	– (2.9)	–

C. Pediatricians[c]

Type of Practice	Direct Hours Worked (in office only)	Visits (in office only)
Solo		
1 worker (RN absent)	31.0	81.5 (2.60)
2 workers (RN absent)	38.0	105.1 (3.03)
3 workers (RN absent)	37.2	110.8 (2.98)
1 worker (RN present)	33.4	93.1 (2.78)
2 workers (RN present)	35.0	108.5 (3.10)
3 workers (RN present)	36.7	131.1 (3.57)
Two-Man Partnership		
2 workers (RN absent)	33.3	91.0 (2.73)

Table 3-4 (cont.)

Type of Practice	Direct Hours Worked (in office only)	Visits (in office only)
3 workers (RN absent)	36.3	113.4 (3.12)
2 workers (RN present)	34.7	112.7 (3.25)
3 workers (RN present)	36.4	116.6 (3.20)
4 workers (RN present)	36.5	123.9 (3.39)
5 workers (RN present)	38.7	127.9 (3.31)
Three-Man Group		
4 workers (RN present)	35.2	108.6 (3.09)
5+ workers (RN present)	38.4	126.1 (3.28)
Four-Man Groups		
5+ workers (RN present)	38.5	115.9 (3.01)
Five or More (Multispecialty) Group		
5+ workers (RN present)	37.3	105.1 (2.82)

D. Hospital Staff Physicians

Field	Direct Hours Worked[d]	Total Hours Worked[e]	Visits[f] Series 1	Visits[f] Series 2
General practice	33	49	135(4.09)	153(4.70)
General surgery	33	59	69(2.09)	86(2.61)
Internal medicine	26	53	52(2.00)	69(2.65)
Pediatricians	21	53	30(1.43)	47(2.24)
All fields	–	50	–	–

[a]Numbers in parentheses in the visits column of section A are the number of visits per hour of patient care (direct hours worked). Weeks worked and expenses correspond to 1969. Hours and visits are for 1970. Source: Center for Health Services Research and Development (1972).

[b]Direct hours per week given in section B of the table are derived from the authors series on direct hours worked in April 1967. Numbers in parentheses are defined as in A. Source: Bailey (1970).

[c]Hours and visits data in section C are for the pediatrician's office. Numbers in parentheses are defined as in A. Data are for October 1967. Source: Yankauer, et al. (1970).

[d]Number of hours full-time hospital staff physicians spent treating patients in the hospital per week during 1966. Source: *Hospital Physician*, July 1967, pp. 35-39.

[e]Number of hours spent in all professional activity per week during 1966, including private practice.

[f]Series 1 in section D is the median number of visits with the physician's own patients in the hospital. Series 2 includes other physicians' patients treated by the physician in addition to his own in the hospital. Numbers in parentheses are visits per direct hours worked.

Output

Table 3-4 also contains a productivity measure, visits per physician hour in patient care. Judging from Part A of the table, partnerships and groups are more productive than solo practices. [The numbers in parentheses in the visits column are visits per direct (patient care) hour.] However, when one disaggregates according to the source of income, it is apparent that fee-for-service practices are far more productive than salary and retainer practices. This data suggests that physician income per unit of extra effort is relatively similar among fee-for-service practice types, but that there are marked differences in incentives between fee-for-service and salary-retainer practices. Unfortunately, the data source does not give standard deviations and sample sizes; thus formal statistical tests for the differences between means cannot be conducted. But the productivity differences by source of income are so pronounced that they are probably significant.

Data on internist and pediatrician productivity by practice size is presented in Parts B and C of Table 3-4. Internist data comes from a study of single specialty groups in the San Francisco Bay Area conducted by Bailey (1968, 1970). Using a visits per physician hour measure, the three-man group is the most productive and the clinic, the least. Unfortunately, Bailey does not describe the method by which the clinic physicians are compensated; thus, it is not possible to determine whether this pattern reflects group size, payment method (fee-for-service vs. salary-capitation) or both.[14]

The evidence on pediatricians in Part C is from a study by Yankauer et al. (1970). Size of group, number of aides per pediatrician, hours, and visits are given in the table. It reveals a pattern similar to Bailey's. Even though the pediatrician-aide ratio is generally higher for the three-, four-, and five-man group than for the two-man partnership, pediatricians in the two-man group are shown to be more productive (with the exception of the two-man partnership—2 workers—RN absent category).[15] Like Bailey, the authors are not explicit about cost- and revenue-sharing arrangements. In any case, the pediatrician data is consistent with that of internists. The differences are far lower than those according to source of income which are presented in Part A.

According to Part D, productivity with the exception of general practitioners, is much lower in salaried hospital practice. Part of the fee-for-service-salaried practice difference may reflect case-mix;[16] data, not currently available on case-mix by method of compensation, is needed before more definitive statements can be made. Nevertheless, comparing Part D with Parts B and C, it would appear that rather marked case-mix differences would be required to explain productivity differences of this magnitude.

Hours and Weeks

Judging from Part A of Table 3-4, solo practitioners work fewer hours per year than do physicians in partnerships, informal associations, and groups. Fee-for-service physicians work substantially longer hours per week than do those on salary or retainer. Bailey's data indicates that internist hours spent in patient care decline as a function of the size of group, but internists in two-man partnerships have longer workweeks than those in solo practice. Bailey's sample size is small, and since no standard deviations are given, it is, as before, not possible to perform statistical tests for differences in means. Data on hours of work from the Yankauer study shows no discernible relationship between physician hours devoted to patient care and group size. Comparing mean hours in Part D with means in the other parts, it is apparent that hospital staff physicians have relatively short workweeks.

Table 3-5 presents evidence on hours and weeks worked by specialty. Almost all the nonsolo means of direct patient care hours are significantly higher than the corresponding solo means in 1965. A similar pattern holds for 1970 although no statistical tests can be performed from these data. In contrast to this evidence on the workweek, Owens (1968) reports *Medical Economics'* findings that solo practitioners spent 4.1 weeks away from their practices as opposed to 4.0 for expense-sharers, and 4.5, 4.4, and 4.6 for two, three, and four to nine physician groups, respectively. Group size may have a different effect on weeks worked than on the length of the workweek.

Although the tables are not definitive, the data presented in this subsection suggests that substantial differences in cost, productivity, and work hours exist between fee-for-service and the salaried practice. Within the fee-for-service category, differences are relatively small. Probably one reason for the small within fee-for-service difference is that larger groups change their incentive structures in order to maintain work incentives for the individual physician.

Physician Choice of Practice Mode

Although evidence on the optimal mode of physician practice is inconclusive, research on the physician's practice mode decision is needed. Once more is known about the relative efficiency and effectiveness of alternative modes, policymakers may want to know how to influence physician choice of practice mode. Also, if there are systematic taste differences among physicians who choose alternative practice types, the measured response of costs, productivity, and work patterns to financial incentives may incorporate substantial biases. For the latter reason, practice mode choice and the impact of incentives on physician performance are related topics.

Table 3-6 gives mean incomes by practice type. Income differences between solo and partnership-group practice have persisted through the mid and late 1960s. Hospital staff and medical school faculty incomes are far lower than those of physicians as a whole. Two-man partnership is reported to be somewhat higher than group income, especially in 1969. Part B of Table 3-6, based on longitudinal data on physicians entering practice in 1962, is very pertinent to

Table 3-5
Hours of Work by Type of Practice and Specialty

Part A—Direct Patient Care Hours, 1965[a]

Specialty	Mean	Standard Deviation	Significant at 1%?	at 5%
General Practice				
Solo (541)	47.2	13.7		
Nonsolo (248)	53.6	11.4	Yes	–
General Surgery				
Solo (405)	43.9	14.2		
Nonsolo (272)	48.2	12.6	Yes	–
Internal Medicine				
Solo (282)	44.0	13.7		
Nonsolo (155)	49.1	11.9	Yes	–
Obstetrics-Gynecology				
Solo (117)	43.2	13.5		
Nonsolo (103)	52.1	12.2	Yes	–
Pediatrics				
Solo (14.3)	44.1	14.3		
Nonsolo (12.2)	49.3	12.2	No	Yes
Psychiatry				
Solo (121)	39.1	9.9		
Nonsolo (21)	32.4	10.5	Yes	–
Radiology				
Solo (21)	30.8	12.5		
Nonsolo (84)	30.2	15.3	–	No
Anesthesiology				
Solo (36)	36.8	14.9		
Nonsolo (79)	45.7	11.8	Yes	–
"Other"				
Solo (71)	37.5	13.0		
Nonsolo (55)	35.5	13.7	–	No

Part B—Direct Patient Care Hours, 1970 and Weeks Worked, 1969[b]

Type of Practice	Specialty				
	General Practice	General Surgery	Internal Medicine	Obstetrics-Gynecology	Pediatrics
Solo	47.0/48.3	46.8/48.0	45.8/48.0	49.2/49.1	47.9/48.8
Two-man partnership	51.8/48.1	50.0/48.2	46.9/48.2	51.0/48.8	51.1/49.0
Informal association	51.4/48.2	45.7/49.0	50.7/46.8	57.7/49.2	48.0/47.8
Group	50.6/48.3	48.9/48.1	50.0/47.6	51.8/48.0	48.0/47.8

[a]Numbers in parentheses are observations. Significance tests are for differences in solo-nonsolo means.

[b]Numbers to the right of the / are weeks worked. Sources: Part A—Theodore and Sutter (1967); Part B—Center for Health Services Research and Development (1972).

this discussion since young physicians may be expected to change practice settings most readily. This data indicates that group is not generally higher than solo physician income in the first five years of practice. Part B refutes the conventional wisdom that group practice is relatively attractive financially to a physician at an initial stage in his career.[17]

A 1969-1970 *Hospital Physician* survey of interns, residents, and fellows is the most complete source on practice mode preferences of physicians.[18] Table 3-7 gives the practice preferences of residents who responded that they were reasonably certain about the type of practice they will enter. Of the 649 residents in the sample, 408 had decided to enter solo, partnership, group hospital practice, or academic medicine. One-hundred-thirty-eight residents either failed to answer the question or stated they were undecided. The remaining physicians preferred fields with comparatively few physicians, such as public health or a combination of modes, for example, academic medicine and private practice. Of particular interest is the small percentage selecting solo practice, slightly over 10 percent.

Factors that residents feel are important considerations in choice of practice mode are revealed in Table 3-8. Only respondents who indicated that they had made a practice mode decision are included. Physicians entering solo practice stress "professional independence" more than others. Yet this factor is also important to future partnership and group physicians. This finding suggests that a large proportion of physicians may not be amenable to yielding much decision making power to the group. A much more intensive study of physician attitudes toward delegation of practice responsibility would be fruitful.

"Income potential" and "financial security" apply to the upper and lower ends of the distribution of physician incomes, respectively. Hospital staff and academic practices are generally considered to be the most secure, but offer the lowest probability of obtaining large incomes. Solo practice is at the opposite end of the spectrum. For this reason, one expects physicians choosing hospital and academic jobs to be the least interested in "income security." The opposite pattern should hold for future solo practitioners. If one compares percentages at the extremes, this pattern holds. 56.3 percent of future hospital staff physicians value "financial security" highly, but only 12.5 percent value "income potential." By contrast only 14.3 percent of the future solo practitioners value "financial security" highly as compared with 32.7 percent for "income potential." Physicians entering group practices stress both approximately equally. This pattern suggests that some physician respondents may consider that both terms apply to mean income rather than its dispersion. If so, income appears to be especially important to future group practitioners. Teaching and research are more important to future hospital staffers and academicians. Regularity of hours matters comparatively more to future group and hospital staff physicians. Goldberg (1969) states that shorter workweek and freedom from night calls are two of the principal advantages of salaried practice. Substantial variation in the percentages presented in Table 3-8 suggests important preference differences among physicians choosing alternative practice modes.

Table 3-6
Physicians' Earnings by Practice Type

Part A – All Physicians

Type of Practice	1965	1966	1967	1968	1969	1970
Solo	$26,680[b]	$29,740[c]	—	$36,899[a]	$39,702[a]	—
Partnership-group	33,430[b]	36,720[c]	—	—	—	—
Two-man partnership	—	—	—	41,740[a]	46,953[a]	—
Informal association	—	—	—	40,533[a]	43,560[a]	—
Group	—	—	—	41,376[a]	43,601[a]	—
Staff	—	—	—	—	—	$25,500[e]
Faculty	—	—	—	—	—	26,700
	—	—	—	—	—	28,100
Total	$28,960	$32,170	$34,730[d]	$37,378[a]	$39,702[a]	$29,600

Part B – Initial Earnings in Private Physician Practice

Field	Earnings Profile of Physicians Entering Practice in 1962									
	1962		1963		1964		1965		1966	
	Solo	Group	Solo	Group	Solo	Group	Solo	Group	Solo	Group

General Practice	$15,434	$12,662	$21,234	$19,723	$27,453	$25,317	$31,651	$27,085	$38,759	$31,115
General Surgery	11,780	12,500	20,117	21,851	29,176	27,075	30,746	29,987	38,759	31,115
Internal Medicine	20,034	12,133	26,403	22,656	28,856	34,570	Not available	Not available	Not available	Not available
Obstetrics-Gynecology	12,426	12,568	20,818	15,232	27,226	20,354	30,593	26,678	37,151	29,568
Pediatrics	$11,945	$12,301	$17,088	$20,649	$22,238	$25,971	Not available	Not available	Not available	Not available

Sources: Part A

aCenter for Health Services Research and Development (1972).

bMedical Economics, June 12 and June 26, 1967.

cMedical Economics, December 11, 1967.

dMedical Economics, May 25, 1970.

eHospital Physician, December 1970. Top and bottom numbers pertain to medical and surgical specialties, respectively.

Source: Part B

Magnan (1967).

Table 3-7

Practice Mode Preferences or Residents When the Decision Is Made[a]

When Selected	Type of Practice Selected					Total Observations by Timing of Education
	Solo	Partnership	Group	Hospital Staff	Academic	
Before medical school	9	6	5	0	5	25
During medical school	8	19	34	11	22	94
During internship	9	13	33	17	7	79
During residency	23	72	60	35	20	210
Total observations by practice mode	49	110	132	63	54	408

[a]Table gives number of observations.

Source: Constructed from *1969-1970 Hospital Physician Survey of Interns, Residents, and Fellows.*

Table 3-9 describes major deterrents to careers in specific types of practices as viewed by the residents who have already made practice mode choices. Irrespective of the mode the respondent has chosen, private practice ranks low on "irregular hours," "danger of lawsuits," and "lack of technical resources." Hospital practice ranks low on "lack of professional independence" and "relatively low income." Academic medicine's principal deterrents are "lack of professional independence," "relatively low income," and "lack of personal contact with patients." "Relatively low income" appears to be somewhat more important to future private practitioners than to the other physicians.

Suggested Research

Much remains to be learned about the structure of incentives in medical practice, how they vary according to group size, and what the effects of alternative incentives on medical practice performance are. If output, price, and input cost decisions are made by individual members, one should expect a loss in efficiency. Fortunately, group decision making seems to become more important as the number of physician members increases. However, more detailed data is needed to verify current impressions. Our knowledge of the effect of incentives will remain quite limited until more specific information is gathered on internal

Table 3-8
Factors Influencing Practice Mode Choice by Type of Practice Selected[a]

| | | Practice Mode Selected | | | |
| | | Private Practice | | | |
Factor	Solo	Partnership	Group	Hospital Staff	Academic
Professional independence	73.5	64.5	48.3	15.6	23.6
Teaching opportunities	6.1	12.7	9.7	37.5	65.5
Income potential	32.7	43.6	41.0	12.5	3.6
Research opportunities	2.0	3.6	3.7	26.6	49.1
Involvement with patients	32.7	46.4	44.8	14.1	10.9
Prestige in community	16.3	16.4	11.9	3.1	9.1
Financial security	14.3	26.4	38.8	20.3	10.9
Regularity of hours	12.2	32.7	51.5	56.3	27.3
Administrative challenge	0.0	1.0	3.0	1.6	3.6
Geographic location	14.2	20.0	29.1	6.3	7.3
Type of medical community	14.2	15.5	26.1	3.1	21.8
Prestige among colleagues	2.0	8.2	3.7	9.4	16.4
Type of patients	26.5	23.6	26.1	3.1	16.4
Technical resources	6.1	6.4	14.9	20.3	23.6
Lack of clerical burden	6.1	6.4	19.4	14.1	9.1
No. of observations	49	110	134	55	64

[a]Percentage answering that factor was of major importance.
Source: Constructed from *1969-1970 Hospital Physician Survey of Interns, Residents, and Fellows.*

incentives in various types of practices as well as on factors leading to physician choices of specific practice modes.

Three specific areas for research are suggested by the analysis presented in this chapter. First, there is a need for research describing how decisions with respect to input purchases, physician effort, and pricing are made in various practice settings. Much of this information can be obtained from direct questions. Researchers have preferred to infer inefficiencies indirectly from empirical cost functions,[19] but the indirect approach gives general indications of inefficiency at best and does not allow one to locate its source. Second, studies of practice mode choices would be useful. To date, there has been no effort to

Table 3-9

Major Deterrents to Careers in Private Practice, Hospital Practice, and Academic Medicine as Viewed by Physicians in Residency Programs[a]

Deterrents	Priv. Pract.[a]			Hosp. Pract.	Academic
	S	P	G		
Irregular hours	59.2	64.5	73.1	59.4	45.5
Lack of prof. independence	0.0	0.1	1.5	1.6	3.6
Relatively low income	0.0	0.1	0.1	0.0	1.8
Financial security	14.3	10.0	9.7	7.8	7.3
Danger of lawsuits	44.9	35.4	38.1	29.6	20.0
Medicare—other programs	18.4	20.9	28.4	25.0	18.2
Paperwork	24.5	27.3	34.3	29.7	14.5
Inadequate patient load	10.2	2.7	1.5	7.8	7.3
Excessive patient load	32.7	31.8	51.5	31.3	25.5
Lack of personal contact with patients	0.0	3.6	3.7	1.6	9.0
Lack of teaching opportunity	57.1	37.3	45.5	37.5	49.1
Lack of research opportunity	46.9	34.5	32.1	39.1	41.8
Type of patients	8.2	5.4	8.2	12.5	16.4
Lack of technical resources	28.6	23.6	26.1	23.4	29.1
Irregular hours	6.1	1.8	5.2	3.1	3.6
Lack of prof. independence	44.9	46.3	44.8	25.0	36.4
Relatively low income	30.6	23.6	32.8	26.5	12.7
Financial security	2.0	6.3	6.7	7.8	1.8
Danger of lawsuits	4.1	8.2	1.5	9.3	3.6
Medicare—other programs	16.3	17.3	20.1	12.5	9.1
Paperwork	24.5	26.4	20.9	15.6	18.2
Inadequate patient load	4.1	9.0	4.5	3.1	1.8
Excessive patient load	22.4	3.6	3.7	18.8	14.5
Lack of personal contact with patients	20.4	15.5	14.9	9.4	9.1
Lack of teaching opportunity	4.1	3.6	3.0	4.7	7.3
Lack of research opportunity	2.0	1.8	3.0	6.3	3.6
Type of patients	24.5	10.9	20.1	3.1	9.1
Lack of technical resources	4.1	2.7	2.2	4.7	0.0
Irregular hours	4.1	0.0	1.0	3.1	5.5
Lack of prof. independence	36.7	39.1	38.1	20.3	20.0
Relatively low income	46.9	60.0	63.4	43.8	6.2
Financial security	16.3	13.6	14.2	7.8	5.5
Danger of lawsuits	0.0	1.0	1.5	3.1	0.0

Table 3-9 (cont.)

Deterrents	Priv. Pract.[a]			Hosp. Pract.	Academic
	S	P	G		
Medicare–other programs	8.2	9.1	7.5	7.8	3.6
Paperwork	16.3	23.6	14.2	17.2	23.6
Inadequate patient load	20.4	25.4	29.9	7.8	7.3
Excessive patient load	4.1	1.0	1.0	1.6	1.8
Lack of personal contact with patients	59.2	54.5	48.5	28.1	21.8
Lack of teaching opportunity	0.0	0.0	0.0	4.7	3.6
Lack of research opportunity	2.0	0.0	0.0	1.6	1.8
Type of patients	10.2	13.6	10.5	1.6	0.0
Lack of technical resources	0.0	1.0	1.0	0.0	0.0

The heading above the Priv. Pract., Hosp. Pract., and Academic columns reads: **Private Practice / Physician Has Chosen**.

Key: S = Solo practice P = Partnership G = Group practice

[a]Percentage answering item is major deterrent.

Source: Constructed from *1969-1970 Hospital Physician Survey of Interns, Residents, and Fellows.*

gather information on preferences for groups of specific sizes. Moreover, available data focuses on practice preferences, but there has been no emphasis on studying characteristics of physicians who made specific practice mode decisions in the recent past. The latter type of analysis may be more fruitful because it is difficult to capture the intensity of practice preferences. The third type of study concerns the effect of the incentives on performance. It would be useful to measure intervening variables as well as output, price, and input costs under alternative incentive structures. For example, what type of information is gathered in alternative practice settings before a major capital purchase is made? Specifically, how does the physician's work schedule change as n increases? In sum, emphasis in future research on this and related issues should be substantially more detailed than it has been to date.

Notes

1. See, for example, United States Department of Health, Education, and Welfare (1967) and Fein (1967).

2. X-efficiency is thought to be important outside the health field as well. For general discussions of the concept, see Leibenstein (1966), Shelton (1967), and Comanor and Leibenstein (1969).

3. Also see Pauly (1970). Olson (1965) discusses the disincentive effects inherent in large groups.

4. That the expression in brackets is negative (except for the trivial case, $q = 0$) is readily seen. $q*$ is determined at the point where marginal revenue equals marginal cost. Given Equations (3.1) and (3.2), this condition is expressed as

$$a_0 + 2a_1 q + a_2 Z = c_1 + c_2 + c_4/n.$$

But $2a_1 q$ is always negative or zero since a_1 is always negative and q, nonnegative. Therefore, without $2a_1 q$, the left side is greater than or equal to the right.

5. If marginal costs vary with scale, probably the most important source of variation is the imputed physician cost. As the physician produces more, the marginal cost associated with his effort may rise. If so, (3.4) becomes

$$q* = 1/(2a_1 - \bar{c}_2) [-a_0 - a_2 Z + c_1 + c_2 + (c_4/n)].$$

where c_2 is the imputed cost coefficient associated with q. The corresponding cost function is

$$c_0 + (c_1 + c_2)q + \bar{c}_2 q^2 + (c_3/n) + (c_4/n)q.$$

This modification would not alter the basic conclusions of the analysis in the text.

6. One way to ascertain the sign of dY/dn is to observe whether physicians have been joining large cost-sharing groups. In a recent paper, Frech and Ginsburg (1973) suggest this approach for the analysis of the relative efficiency of various organizational forms of medical practice. If a particular practice mode is becoming more prevalent, it is then judged to provide a better means for satisfying physicians' preferences. Thus, it is seen to be more efficient overall in the private if not from the social vantage point. A major difficulty with this method is that many factors change simultaneously, and changes in the prevalence of various organizational forms do not represent movement to a single (static) equilibrium state. For example, a group may grow relative to solo practice because the population is becoming increasingly urbanized. The trend might not have occurred in the absence of these demographic changes. For the Frech-Ginsburg approach to yield useful evidence, one would have to demonstrate that all factors other than the relative efficiency of various modes were held constant. Research methods suggested in the last section of this chapter are preferable.

7. There is surprisingly little evidence on this point. Rorem (1931) reports considerable variability in group fee-setting practices, but his information is for

the late 1920s. Papers, such as Weinerman (1969), stress that individual members function quite independently. But Weinerman's statement is with reference to peer review within the group, not pricing.

8. If c_2 depends in part on the physician's expected income and these expectations are based on income received in the recent past, an exceptionally profitable year would be followed by one in which each member sought to restrict output. If the physician bases effort on current income which includes a share of the net return from other group members, the analysis becomes more complex, since this introduces interaction among group members in output and price decisions. However, it is probably difficult for the individual member to judge the current contribution of others to group profits; the individual physician probably projects current group profits on the basis of past experience to a considerable extent.

9. Senior members of groups often receive a larger share of group profits.

10. The reason for the emphasis on "may" is that optimal output involves a corner solution if no bonus condition on effort is offered, and small or moderate salary incentives may not move physicians from the corner.

11. A minor difference may exist to the extent that the minimum effort required per prepayment MD may vary with the ratio of subscribers to physicians.

12. *Medical Economics'* (ME) "Continuing Survey" typically specifies a separate category for expense-sharers. The American Medical Association's "Periodic Survey of Physicians" does not. ME's data contains no information related to the institutional structure of practice, but does describe practice costs, fees, income, and output.

13. As stated above, this scheme reduces to cost-sharing if revenues are apportioned precisely according to the amount of revenue attributable to each member, and the same is not true of costs.

14. The data in Parts B and C are comparable to those for internists and pediatricians given in Altman et al. (1965) and Bergman et al. (1966), respectively.

15. The fact that four- and five-man aide categories are open-ended reinforces the statement that productivity in the largest group declines.

16. Discussion in the *Hospital Physician* which accompanies this data indicates that hospital physicians treat more difficult, referral cases.

17. *Medical Economics'* data given in Jeffers (1967) shows that partnership-group initial incomes are higher in some, but not in all specialties. Jeffers' data is for 1965.

18. This section draws substantially from Sloan (1973).

19. For example, Newhouse (1973) and Yett (1967).

Bibliography

Altman, I.; H. Kroeger; D. Clarke; A. Johnson; and C. Shepa, "The Office Practice of Internists, II. Patient Load," *Journal of the American Medical Association*, Vol. 193: 667-72 (August 23, 1965).

Bailey, R.M., "A Comparison of Internists in Solo and Fee-for-Service Group Practice in the San Francisco Bay Area," *Bulletin of the New York Academy of Medicine*, Vol. 44: 1293-1303 (November 1968).

_____, "Economies of Scale in Medical Practice," in *Empirical Studies in Health Economies*, edited by Herbert E. Klarman. Baltimore: The Johns Hopkins Press, 1970.

Balfe, B.E., and M.E. McNamara, *Survey of Medical Groups in the U.S.*. Chicago: American Medical Association, 1968.

Bergman, A.; S. Dassel; and R. Wedgwood, "Time-Motion Study of Practicing Pediatricians," *Pediatrics*, Vol. 38: 254-63 (August 1966).

Center for Health Services Research and Development, American Medical Association, *The Profile of Medical Practice, 1972*. Chicago: American Medical Association, 1972.

Comanor, W.S., and H. Leibenstein, "Allocative Efficiency, X-Efficiency and the Measurement of Welfare Losses," *Economica*, Vol. 36: 304-9 (August 1969).

Fein, R., *The Doctor Shortage*. Washington: The Brookings Institution, 1967.

Frech, H.E., and P.B. Ginsburg, "Optimal Scale in Group Medical Practice: A Survivor Analysis," Michigan State University Working Paper, 1973.

Goldberg, J., "The Security of Salary Practice: Who Needs It," *Hospital Physician*, pp. 67-69 (February 1969).

Hunt, G.H., and M.S. Goldstein, *Medical Group Practice in the United States*. Washington: U.S. Government Printing Office, Public Health Service Pub. No. 77, 1951.

Jeffers, W.N., "Compare Earnings with Your Age Group's," *Medical Economics*, pp. 85-9 (August 7, 1967).

Leibenstein, H., "Allocative Efficiency vs. 'X-Efficiency'," *American Economic Review*, Vol. 56: 392-415 (June 1966).

Magnan, W.F., "Instant Success for Young Practitioners?" *Hospital Physician*, pp. 56-61 (December 1967).

Newhouse, J., "The Economics of Group Practice," *Journal of Human Resources*, Vol. 8: 37-56 (Winter 1973).

Olson, M., *The Logic of Collective Action*. Cambridge, Mass.: Harvard University Press, 1965.

Pauly, M.V., "Efficiency, Incentives and Reimbursement for Health Care," *Inquiry*, Vol. 7: 114-31 (March 1970).

Rorem, C.R., *Private Group Clinics*. Chicago: University of Chicago Press, 1931.

Shelton, J.P., "Allocative vs. 'X-Efficiency': Comment," *American Economic Review*, Vol. 57: 1252-58 (December 1967).

Sloan, F., *Planning Public Expenditures on Mental Health Service Delivery*. Santa Monica, Cal.: Rand Corporation RM-6339-NYC, 1971.

_____ , *Supply Responses of Young Physicians: An Analysis of Physicians in Residency Programs*. Santa Monica, Cal.: Rand Corporation R-1131-OEO, 1973.

Taylor, V., and J. Newhouse, *Ambulatory Care at the Good Samaritan Medical Center*. Santa Monica, Cal.: Rand Corporation RM-6342-GS, 1970.

Theodore, C.N., and G.E. Sutter, "A Report of the First Periodic Survey of Physicians," *Journal of the American Medical Association*, Vol. 202: 516-24 (November 6, 1967).

Todd, C., and M.E. McNamara, *Survey of Medical Groups in the United States, 1969*. Chicago: American Medical Association, 1971.

United States Department of Health, Education, and Welfare, *A Report to the President on Medical Care Prices*. Washington: U.S. Government Printing Office, 1967.

United States Public Health Service, *Medical Groups in the United States, 1959*. Washington: U.S. Government Printing Office, Public Health Service Pub. No. 1063, 1963.

Weinerman, R., "Problems and Perspectives in Group Practice," *Group Practice*, Vol. 18: 27-33 (April 1969).

Yankauer, A.; J.P. Connelly; and J.J. Feldman, "Physician Productivity in the Delivery of Ambulatory Care," *Medical Care*, Vol. 8: 35-46 (January/February 1970).

Yett, D.E., "An Evaluation of Alternative Methods of Estimating Physician's Expenses Relative to Output," *Inquiry*, Vol. 4: 3-27 (March 1967).

Patient Participation and Productivity in the Medical Care Sector

Fredrick L. Golladay*

Introduction

Attempts to increase the productivity of the medical care system are commonly couched in terms of efforts to transfer responsibility for parts of patient care from physicians to more specialized, paraprofessional health workers. Implicit in this approach is the notion that the functions of the health care system have been properly defined historically. However, a relatively unexplored device for reducing the burden on health care resources is patient participation in care. The growth in consumer sophistication and parallel developments in diagnosis and treatment suggest that a more efficient utilization of the formal health care system is possible, by means of direct replacement of professional providers by patients or their families.

A reappraisal of the roles of the patient and the professional provider in responding to health care problems is important in the development of new health professions. The physician extenders—the physician assistant and the nurse practitioner—are being promoted largely as substitutes for physicians in routine, uncomplicated care. The modest training requirements for these extenders suggest that at least some of the activities being delegated to them could also be performed by patients with small amounts of specific education. However, although a large number of anecdotal accounts of patient classification, self-care, patient compliance, and health consumerism have suggested that increased patient involvement is desirable, these studies have generally reflected the narrow perspective of their authors—as health educators, hospital administrators, or nurses. As a result, patient participation in health care delivery remains a relatively unexplored device for affecting productivity of the system.

The purpose of this chapter therefore is to synthesize previous research on the patient's role in health care delivery and to indicate appropriate directions for future research.

The literature review is of course not exhaustive, but it does attempt to identify the more seminal works. It draws from the major bibliographical sources and from the more recent journals in health education, nursing and public health, and also from the journals in primary care. The review includes work on

*Economist, Development Economics Department, International Bank for Reconstruction and Development.

effects of patient participation on health status, health maintenance activities, compliance, utilization, self-care, effects of patient knowledge, and educational strategies.

It should be noted at the outset that "patient participation" will be rather broadly defined. The term will be taken to mean not only direct involvement in the production of psychomotor tasks by patients, but also by members of their households, and will also include participation in choosing levels of utilization, phasing treatments, monitoring and evaluating therapy, and organizing and executing programs of health maintenance.

Effects on Health Status

The notion of health status has no universally accepted operational definition. The literature on the impact of health care on health status is consequently not well unified. Extensive biomedical and clinical research supports the view that specific programs of prevention or treatment appear to suppress or remedy specific complaints. Rather than attempt to exhaust this literature, we shall simply note its existence. Most, if not all, common procedures or practices are supported by some medical research. The literature on medical practice focuses on the medical implications of treatments—particularly with respect to side effects and complications—to the exclusion of issues of productivity or cost-effectiveness; there have been very few formal attempts to assess the economic efficiency of alternative modes of care. The rather superficial literature on the HMO concept suggests that preventive care and early diagnosis are preferable to epidemic care. This conclusion has been drawn from analyses of the performances of the Health Plan of Greater New York and of the Kaiser-Permanente System,[1] but these studies were based upon aggregate outcome data and provide minimal insights into either the total program of care being purchased by participants or the processes by which these organizations reduce the cost of care.

We note here that the question of which health services should be produced in greater quantities in order to improve health status has not been answered. Several researchers have sought to evaluate particular procedures or practices, and the more important of these contributions are reviewed below.

Health Maintenance Activities

Preventive care has been a major focus of evaluative research. Several studies have examined the usefulness of periodic examinations. Franco et al. (1961), in a panel study of salaried employees of Consolidated Edison Company of New York, found that major disease was discovered over a ten year period in asymptomatic form in 59 percent of those examined. David (1961), however, questions the contribution of such examinations to the reduction of disability or mortality. Wade et al. (1964), conclude from analyses of medical records for a group of 765 employed males that disabling diseases were diagnosed frequently in the course of periodic examinations; they did not demonstrate, however, that early diagnosis increased the effectiveness of treatment. Grinaldi (1965), in an analysis of matched groups of employees of the General Electric Company, established that the costs of medical care for the group not being examined exceeded that of the experimental group by more than the cost of the periodic examination.[2]

The value of innoculations in preventing communicable diseases is accepted. The literature of public health and health education abound with descriptions of programs to induce people to participate in innoculation programs (several of which are reviewed below). Similarly, the efficacy of early diagnosis of cancer, cardio-vascular disease, tuberculosis and dental problems has motivated efforts to identify risk factors and signs and to encourage self diagnosis. The accompanying research has examined both the value of early decision and methods of insuring early identification of problems.

Compliance with Medical Treatment

The effectiveness of the health care system in improving health status is widely thought to be eroded by noncompliant patients, and considerable research has focused upon the noncompliance of patients with regimens of treatment. Presumably, a part of noncompliance may be attributed to ignorance of the significance of instructions or of the underlying rationale for prescriptions. Curtis (1961) and Schwartz et al. (1962) investigated the compliance of elderly, ambulatory patients with programs of chemotherapy and found that more than 60 percent of patients were noncompliant. The patients omitted medications, relied upon self medication with unprescribed drugs, obtained incorrect dosages, and improperly timed or sequenced drugs. The researchers did not seek to evaluate the impact of noncompliance on the efficacy of treatment nor did they report their results in such a way as to permit interpretation of the seriousness of noncompliance. In a follow-up study of domiciliary tuberculosis patients, Pragoff (1962) found that only one-fourth of the population was noncompliant with drug therapy, but that more than three-fifths were violating instructions regarding diet and activity restrictions. Several studies have revealed that noncompliance is most serious with nonpainful, chronic disease. Preston and Miller (1964) evaluated compliance by chemical analysis of urine samples and concluded that noncompliance was in part a result of lack of confidence in the therapeutic value of the treatment, and advocated greater emphasis on the education of patients in the rationale for the treatment. Davis (1966) has summarized the literature on patient compliance; he found that 15-93 percent of patients deviate from regimens and that in most studies more than a third of patients were noncompliant.

Attempts to explain noncompliant behavior have focused upon self concept, role definition, and fear of loss of activity as major determinants. Most of the research has been descriptive rather than analytic. Johannsen (1966) found that unskilled workers were particularly likely to violate restrictions on diet and activities. Berkowitz, et al. (1963) examined physicians' perceptions of compliance and concluded from the data that patients who were managing their own conditions were least compliant, suggesting the need for both greater supervision and improved education.

The state of the literature is summarized by Simonds (1966):

We are only beginning to understand the problem of patient compliance with medical regimens and some of the related motivational factors. We know that the beliefs the individual holds . . . are strong influencers of action. We know from the work of several social psychologists that beliefs about the medical condition itself and the effectiveness of available courses of preventive or therapeutic actions are significant variables. These beliefs differ between men as contrasted with women; among young people as contrasted with older people; and among people who have different diseases or feel they might get different diseases. . . . Available research suggests only that these beliefs tend to be associated with actions reported by the patient. Whether they are causative influencers and, even more important, whether they can be effectively manipulated in the form of educational messages to influence behavior is still largely unknown.

Utilization of the Health Care System

The utilization of the formal health care system has been a major subject of concern. Researchers have sought to explain delays in seeking intervention rather than to examine overutilization. The perspective of this research literature is conspicuously noneconomic; the issues of appropriateness of intervention or of optimal timing of intervention are rarely addressed. It is not obvious, however, that it is either necessary or efficient to seek professional assistance for specified conditions. Furthermore, it is not apparent when intervention is appropriate; preventive measures or early diagnosis may not be cost-effective modes of approaching a particular problem.

The willingness of prospective patients to assume a *sick role* as a major determinant of utilization has been the focus of research by Mechanic (1962), Blackwell (1964), and others.[3] Implicit in this work are the notions that the appropriate posture for the sick is one of dependency, and that early treatment is optimal. This tradition of research has emphasized the need to perceive oneself as sick, to seek intervention, to transfer responsibility to a physician, and finally to relinquish the patient role at recovery.

Research has focused upon the variables which correlate with willingness to initiate each of these steps and it has been found that psychosocial problems were less readily presented, that ethnicity affected utilization, and that attitudes toward authority and previous experiences with physicians influenced willingness to seek help. Strikingly, the importance of patient ignorance of medical problems is rarely considered; this is probably a reflection of the research strategy being employed rather than a judgment regarding the role of knowledge.

The growing literature on screening and on preventive health education reviewed above suggests the need for more knowledge and information in order to improve the efficiency with which the health care system is being utilized. The important question of whether utilization levels *should* be increased has not been systematically addressed, however.

Patient Self-Care

Some of the most impressive work on patient participation has examined the potential for increasing patient responsibility for his own care. A number of demonstration projects for the care of the chronically ill have illustrated this notion. The need for continuous management of diabetes, chronic heart disease and tuberculosis in particular, has suggested that it would be cost-effective to transfer some responsibilities to the patient or his family. Self-care programs for diabetes are the most widespread. Systematic curricula on diet, self diagnosis, and chemotherapy have been initiated; the literature reports numerous programs. An excellent example is found in the Charles T. Miller Hospital, St. Paul, Minnesota.[4] Home dialysis for kidney patients has been introduced by Peter Bent Brigham Hospital in Boston in order to reduce the cost of care; a plan of instruction has been initiated which permits transfer of responsibility for care to members of the patients family (O'Neill, 1971; Merrill et al., 1964). A program of patient education for heart patients, conducted by the New Jersey Department of Health, illustrated the potential contributions of activated patients. The group was interested in the development of the disease, medication, diet and treatment. An experimental evaluation of the program revealed that the study group required approximately one-third as many hospital admissions and one-fourth as many days of hospital care. Readmissions were less than half of the control group average for the study group. Direct measures of compliance and health status also revealed the substantial superiority of the study group (Rosenberg, 1971).

The University of Kentucky Medical Center's care-by-parent unit provides an interesting counterpoint to the programs of patient intervention for chronic diseases described above. The unit employs mothers of hospitalized children to provide routine care and maintenance. The program was motivated by both economic considerations and the need to reduce the psychological trauma of hospitalization for pediatric patients. The hospital rooms were designed to permit the parent to live in and a utility room provided for food preparation and housekeeping. The parent is supervised by the medical staff. The cost of hospitalization in the unit is approximately 60 percent of that in the pediatric ward. Direct personnel costs are reduced from $10.31 a day to $3.81 (James and Wheeler, 1964).

This review suggests that the economic as well as psychic benefits from patient participation in care would be substantial. Much of the literature is casual in discussing the economic or even health status implications of participation, but wherever the issue has been addressed, the gains have been shown to be large. The major unresolved issue is whether professional intervention is essential for a large number of medical conditions, but the potential for involving the patient in care ought to be further examined.

Effects of Patient Knowledge

The next topic to consider is whether desirable changes in patient behavior can be expected to result from increases or improvements in patient knowledge. A number of studies have sought to evaluate the level of health knowledge held by the lay public through direct interview or questionnaires; others have examined the perceptions of physicians and pharmacists of the level of lay knowledge. Researchers conclude that a large discrepancy exists between acknowledged health care needs and utilization, that patients frequently hold beliefs which are contradictory to diagnostic and treatment procedures, and that few hold a preventive view of disease (Feldman, 1966; Kirscht, et al., 1966).

A number of studies have examined the beliefs and knowledge of the public regarding specific diseases. Much of this literature focuses on highly communicable and on chronic illnesses. Studies of tuberculosis suggest that the public is fairly well informed regarding the causes, communicability, diagnosis, and treatment of the disease (Southworth, 1965; Reinstein, 1964). Certain populations were found to be poorly informed, however. The elderly, poor, and low skilled were discovered to be least knowledgeable. Several attempts to identify the target population for an educational campaign and to devise a responsive program have emerged; similar conclusions have been drawn in studies of innoculation for smallpox (Creighton, 1961; Bharara, 1961).

Research on knowledge of cancer and the value of early detection suggests that the asymptomic is indifferent to utilization of early detection, that most persons depend upon their physicians rather than self-initiating tests and that fear has little effect on willingness to obtain tests. The importance of evaluation of apparently healthy persons is not widely acknowledged (American Cancer Society, 1966; Miyaska et al., 1965; Kegeles et al., 1965).

The literature indicates that even for common and highly publicized problems, public beliefs and attitudes are inconsistent with either a preventive mode of care or early detection. Although this problem is most profound among the lower socioeconomic and educational strata, it is widespread. An extensive literature on patient knowledge, beliefs, and attitudes is included in the bibliography.

Educational Strategies for Patients

There exists a massive literature on strategies of patient education. The bulk of this writing draws heavily upon the largely speculative work of educators such as Bruner, Gagne, and Bloom.[5] A more productive branch of the literature seeks to identify appropriate methods of instruction for selected subgroups of patients. The teaching of patients is complicated by the diversity of prior health knowledge, of educational background, and of motivation. Since the most serious problems of patient ignorance appear to be in the least teachable subgroups, this set of issues is very important. The magnitude of this problem is portrayed vividly in a set of anecdotal accounts of patient learning presented by Slowie (1971). She contrasts the teaching challenge in dealing with a young college professor, a retired, illiterate porter, a middle-aged career woman, a pharmacist and a traveling salesman. Hallburg (1970) emphasizes the need to individualize instruction to accommodate learning differences and prior knowledge.

Two distinct traditions in patient education have emerged in the literature. The larger tradition advocates formal educational programs. The second tradition emphasizes the opportunities for informal instruction in parallel with professional care. Here we review the major contributions to these literatures in order to suggest the feasibility and costs of instruction.

The literature on formal instruction is reviewed by Young in a recent *Health Education Monograph* (1967). She equates instruction with communication, then examines alternative modes of communication. Films, posters, programmed instruction, television and group methods are reviewed. Much of the research cited is speculative (or "theoretical") in nature and provided little insight into current practice or potentialities. The problem in motivating learning and in determining readiness for instruction are acknowledged, however.

Several authors have investigated the impact of printed pamphlets on patients' understanding of medical problems. About 75,000 different pamphlets are currently available. Very little evaluation of these materials has been undertaken. It is apparent, however, that they are not profoundly affecting patient attitudes or beliefs, probably because they are not well adapted to the learning needs of the individual patient.[6]

A number of hospitals have developed special, educational programs for groups of patients. These programs have generally been devoted to chronic illnesses or child care for new mothers. A variety of group teaching methods has been employed, including television, films, lectures, and group discussions. These group teaching strategies have frequently been frustrated by the diversity of learning problems represented by each class (Creighton and Gabrielle, 1961). The published literature on these efforts is anecdotal and is not evaluative in perspective. The accounts strongly suggest, however, that adapting a curriculum to the patient is very difficult.[7]

The most appealing approaches to the problems of patient education have emphasized individualization and informal instruction. The diversity of levels of prior knowledge, discipline, and learning abilities that are obtained in a patient population underscores the need to adapt materials to the individual. Several writers have urged that patient needs be assessed as a first step in education.[8] The instruction of the patient might then be conducted in parallel with diagnosis and treatment. Nursing has been the most vigorous in advancing this approach. Cross and Parsons (1971) and Aiken (1970) have emphasized the opportunities afforded by routine nursing activities for discussing diagnosis treatment and rehabilitation. Renner at the University of Wisconsin Family Practice Clinic has stressed the potential for teaching over routine parts of office visits. The advantages of integrating treatment and teaching include, in addition to individualization, opportunities to exploit the motivation to learn what accompanies a problem and economies in the use of staff.[9] It is estimated that substantial teaching is possible at zero marginal cost.

Summary

This survey of the literature on patient participation in the health care system, while suggestive, does not provide a rigorous basis for policy decisions. Thus, in this chapter we draw only tentative conclusions, but these views are suggestive of needed research. The conclusions are derived from a model of patient participation which is incomplete and contrived; hence they should be tempered with expert judgment and caution.

The prior research suggests that the role of the patient in the delivery of health care should be substantially increased; the patient or his family should be induced to pursue preventive rather than episodic care. Although the literature is extremely vague about the gains from preventive care, it is widely presumed that health status would be increased and costs of care reduced if greater reliance were placed on health maintenance. Research on patient compliance indicates that the well intentioned prescriptions of health professionals are frequently subverted by patients. Studies of compliance fail, however, to provide much insight into the significance of noncompliance for health status on the system's productivity in terms of outcomes. Although more than half of the patients have been found to ignore or violate prescribed treatments, the precise nature of the noncompliance and its implications for the health of the patient have not been assessed. Finally, this survey indicates that in selected areas in which pilot programs have been initiated, patient self-care has been successful in both reducing the costs of care and improving the sociopsychological welfare of patients. Pediatric patients in particular have been shown to be responsive to care-by-parents as opposed to professional care.

In those instances in which the economic implications of patient education or self-care have been evaluated, substantial cost reductions have been reported. The direct costs of hospital based care have been reduced by as much as 60 percent, while readmissions have dropped by up to 75 percent. It is of course inappropriate to generalize from these idiosyncratic experiments to the universe of health care, but such pilot studies indicate that the magnitude of economic gains is potentially large.

The impact of overt patient education on the ability or willingness of patients to resort to health maintenance and self-care is ambiguous. Prior research seems to suggest that motivating preventive care is difficult particularly among the apparently able-bodied. The research literature on the utilization of the system does not indicate the importance of ignorance in this problem; rather it focuses on the correlates of willingness to assume a sick role. It is impossible to reject the notion that a clear understanding of the potential value of preventive care would increase utilization of health maintenance services, on the basis of existing research. The interpretive prose which accompanies studies of patient compliance strongly suggests that patient knowledge is a substantial barrier to effective use of the health care system for episodic care. Patients are noted to hold attitudes and beliefs which are inconsistent with regimens of treatment, particularly chemotherapy. The major exception to this set of generalizations is that violations of restrictions of activities appear to be responsive to socioeconomic factors rather than ignorance. Unskilled and poorly educated males in particular reject activity restrictions.

The more impressive experiments in patient participation have been concentrated in areas of chronic disease. Diabetes, kidney failure, and cardiovascular disease have been successfully dealt with through patient participation. This concentration of interest in chronic problems clearly reflects the fact that the stream of benefits from activating the patient is lengthy. A parallel concern for short-term episodic problems would only be appropriate if the costs of activating the patient were very modest. One concludes that focusing attention and resources on patient participation in the management of chronic problems is cost-effective. The role of the patient in other areas of health care is much less obvious.

The development of methods of patient education is rather primitive. It is clear that the ease with which patients can be trained to assume the management of problems varies greatly. The need to devise individualized programs of instruction and to motivate learning strongly argues for careful evaluation of learning needs and tailoring of the content of any curriculum. The overlaying of professional care and patient teaching is a partial solution to these problems. This implies a distinctive mode of medical practice in which providers assume a substantial teaching role.

In summary, a review of prior research on health care and health education suggests that more patient participation in care is cost-effective. The literature does not provide sufficiently detailed analyses to support strongly worded, specific conclusions. Support of health maintenance education, self-care for the chronically ill, and for patient teaching is warranted, however.

Suggested Research

It has already been observed that review of the research literature on patient participation does not provide the complete, systematic view of the subject that one might like to have for recommending policy. In this final section, we identify research topics which would strengthen policy analyses, and we indicate some priorities for research.

Three major research thrusts are required if the economic implications of patient participation in health care are to be assessed systematically. First, the areas of desirable behavioral change must be identified. Second, the determinants of behavior must be ascertained. And third, effective programs for affecting behavioral changes through the determinants of behavior must be developed and evaluated. There appears a priori to be considerable independence among health problems with respect to each of these issues, which suggests that each major category of health problem might be considered independently of other problems.

The first thrust proposed here would seek to identify potentially cost-effective modes of patient participation. These modes are of three types: (1) health maintenance, (2) compliance, and (3) self-care. The notion of health maintenance, although intuitively appealing, has not been subjected to serious economic analysis. It would be useful to evaluate the optimal level of health maintenance as opposed to episodic care and the sensitivity of solution values to the prices of medical services and the opportunity cost of patient supplied inputs. Such an investigation would compare the cost-effectiveness of preventive care and early diagnosis with that of treatment of symptomic conditions, and assess their effects upon productivity in the health care system. It is not obvious, given the costs of prevention or screening, that preventive modes are superior to episodic modes of care. Resolution of this issue would both indicate areas in which patient education is potentially productive and provide insights into the role of health maintenance activities in reducing the cost of medical care. An incidental outcome would be an indication of the optimal periodicity for screening and asymptomic diagnosis. The proposed analysis obviously must distinguish patient strata wherever risk factors can be identified.

The second research effort would focus on the problem of noncompliance. The existing literature documents the extent of noncompliance but fails to either indicate the urgency of the misbehavior or to identify its correlates. It would be useful to know whether noncompliance is a genuine problem in the management of conditions or merely an affront to the provider. Furthermore, if patient education is to be evaluated as an instrument for effecting greater compliance, it is necessary to determine the reasons for noncompliance. The literature suggests that ignorance and misinformation are major sources of the problem but provides little systematic defense for the view. Two sets of studies are therefore proposed. The first would attend the investigations of compliance studies to evaluate the impact of specific types of noncompliance of the effectiveness of professional care. The second would examine the determinants, as opposed to the correlates, of noncompliance; in particular, it would seek to go behind socioeconomic identifiers in an attempt to isolate attitudes or beliefs which produce noncompliant behavior.

The third research effort would investigate cost-effective methods of patient education in both hospital and outpatient settings. The existing literature on the pedagogy of health education is largely anecdotal. It is proposed that a cost-effectiveness type of evaluative research be initiated in order to determine whether education is a viable method for confronting health problems. This research should recognize the differences in learning abilities, language usage, and intellectual backgrounds of strata of patients in order to tailor educational experiences to individuals and hence to increase learning effectiveness. It is likely that much of the proposed analysis could rely upon existing operational programs of health education and participation for data.

Finally, a professional reassessment of the role of the patient in self-care would be useful. It seems likely that a careful review of opportunities for delegation of tasks to patients or patients' households would be suggestive of new modes of care. This exercise seems particularly appropriate in the face of widespread interest in the introduction of new paraprofessions into the health care team: the notion that persons with limited formal training should be delegated some responsibilities previously reserved by the physician suggests that patients might be delegated some of these functions as well.

Notes

1. For discussion of these issues see Herbert Klarman, "Analysis of the HMO Proposal—Its Assumptions, Implications, and Prospects," Health Maintenance Organization: A Reconfiguration of the Health Services Proceedings of the 13th Annual Symposium on Hospital Affairs, May 1971, Graduate Program in Hospital Administration and the Center for Health Administration Studies, Graduate School of Business, University of Chicago, pp. 24-38.

2. See also Siegel (1963) for an extensive bibliography on studies of the effectiveness of periodic examinations.

3. See, specifically, Schulman and Smith (1963) and Phillips (1965).

4. For details, see Ulrich and Kelley (1972).

5. For example, see Slowie (1971).

6. For a review of this literature, see Whealy and Wake (1961).

7. For a cross-sectional view of hospital-based patient education, see Spiegel and Buis (1963), Painton (1964), Green and Durocher (1965), and Meadows (1965).

8. For example, see Ulrich and Kelley (1972).

9. In conversations with the author.

Bibliography

General Studies

Aiken, Linda Harmen, "Patient Problems Are Problems of Learning," *American Journal of Nursing*, Vol. 70, No. 9 (1970).

Davis, James A., *Education for Positive Mental Health*. Chicago: Aldine Publishing Co., 1966.

De la Vega, Marguerite, "New Focus on the Hospital as a Health Center," *Hospitals*, Vol. 40, No. 14 (1966).

Galiher, Claudia B.; Jack Needleman; and Anne J. Rolfe, "Consumer Participation," *HSMHA Health Reports*, Vol. 86, No. 2 (1971).

Hochbaum, Godfrey M., "Research to Improve Health Education," *International Journal of Health Education*, Vol. 8, No. 3 (1965).

Joint Committee on Health Problems in Education of the A.M.A. and N.E.A., *Why Health Education?* Chicago: American Medical Association, 1965.

Klein, Susan F., "Toward a Framework for Evaluating Health Education Activities of a Family Planning Program," *American Journal of Public Health*, Vol. 61, No. 6 (1971).

Nickerson, Hiram H., *Health Education in Occupational Settings*, Boston, Mass.: Medical Foundation, Monograph No. 5, March 1966.

Ozarin, Lucy D., and Claudewell S. Thomas, "Advocacy in Community Mental Health Programs," *American Journal of Public Health*, Vol. 62 No. 4 (1972).

Roberts, Beryl J. (Ed.), *Health Education in Medical Care: Needs and Opportunities*. University of California (Berkeley), School of Public Health, Health Education Division, 1962.

Simonds, Scott K., "Health Education and Medical Care: Focus on the Patient," *Health Education Monographs*, No. 16 (1963).

_____ , "Patient Education Vital, But More Research Need," *Geriatrics* (August 1971).

_____ , "Motivation and Health Insurance," *Proceedings of Second National Conference on Health Education*, Chicago: The American Medical Association, 1966.

Tryoler, Herman A., et al., "Patterns of Preventive Health Behavior in Populations," *Journal of Health and Human Behavior*, Vol. 6, No. 3 (1965).

Ulrich, Marian R., and Kenneth M. Kelley, "Patient Care Includes Teaching: Health Education Department Coordinates Multidisciplinary Programs," *Hospitals*, Vol. 46 (1972).

U.S. Department of Health, Education, and Welfare, Public Health Service, Advisory Committee on Health Education and Communication to the Bureau of State Services, *Education for Health*, Washington, D.C.: U.S. Government Printing Office, Public Health Service Publication No. 1430 (February 1966).

Wegman, Myron E., "Educational Implications for Health Workers and the Public," *Archives of Environmental Health*, Vol. 18 (1969).

Wooden, Howard E., "The Inseparability of Education and Patient Care," in *Health Education in the Hospital*. Chicago: American Hospital Association, 1965.

World Health Organization, PAHO/WHO Inter-Regional Conference on the Postgraduate Preparation of Health Workers for Health Education, *Preparation of Health Workers for Health Education*. Geneva, Switzerland: WHO, Technical Report Series, No. 278, 1964.

Young, Marjorie A.C., et al., "Review of Research Related to Health Education Practice," *Health Education Monographs*, Supplement No. 1 (1963).

Effectiveness of Education–Induced Health Practices

Blackwell, Barbara, "The Literature of Delay in Seeking Medical Care for Chronic Illness," *Health Education Monographs*, No. 16 (1963).

Bruce, Sylvia J., "Do Prenatal Educational Programs Really Prepare for Parenthood?" *Hospital Topics*, Vol. 43, No. 11 (1965).

Dalzell, Irene, "Evaluation of a Prenatal Teaching Program," *Nursing Research*, Vol. 14, No. 2 (1965).

David, W.D., "The Usefulness of Periodic Health Examinations," *Archives of Environmental Health*, Vol. 2, No. 3 (1961).

Eichhorn, Robert L., and Ronald M. Andersen, "Changes in Personal Adjustment to Perceived and Medically Established Heart Disease: A Panel Study," *Journal of Health and Human Behavior*, Vol. 3, No. 4 (1962).

Elsom, K.A., and K.O. Elsom, "The Periodic Health Examination–A Study of Private Practitioners' Attitudes," *Archives of Environmental Health*, Vol. 3, No. 2 (1961).

Franco, S.C., et al., "Periodic Health Examinations: A Long Term Study, 1949-59," *Journal of Occupational Medicine*, Vol. 3, No. 1 (1961).

Gottlieb, Stanley, and Herbert Kramer, "Compliance with Recommendations Following Executive Health Examinations," *Journal of Occupational Medicine*, Vol. 4, No. 12 (1962).

Griffiths, William, "Achieving Change in Health Practices," *Health Education Monographs*, No. 20 (1965).

Grinaldi, John V., "The Worth of Occupational Health Programs: A New Evaluation of Periodic Physical Examinations," *Journal of Occupational Medicine*, Vol. 7, No. 8 (1965).

Hochbaum, Godfrey M., "Learning and Behavior–Alcohol Education for What?" in *Alcohol Education*. U.S. Department of Health, Education, and Welfare, March 1966.

Kerr, Willard A., "Motivation of People," in *Proceedings of First National Conference on Health Education Goals*. Chicago: American Medical Association, 1965.

Klerman, Lorraine V., "Health Education in Industry—Potential and Practice," *Industrial Medicine and Surgery*, Vol. 34, No. 7 (1965).

Rosenstock, Irwin M., "Public Response to Cancer Screening and Detection Programs," *Journal of Chronic Disease*, Vol. 16, No. 5 (1963).

Schonfield, Jacob, et al., "Medical Attitudes and Practices of Parents Toward a Mass Tuberculin-Testing Program," *American Journal of Public Health*, Vol. 53, No. 5 (1963).

Schor, Stanley S., et al., "An Evaluation of the Periodic Health Examination," *Annals of Internal Medicine*, Vol. 61, No. 6 (1964).

Siegel, Gordon S., *Periodic Health Examinations—Abstracts from the Literature*, U.S. Department of Health, Education, and Welfare, Public Health Service, Division of Chronic Disease. Washington, D.C.: U.S. Government Printing Office, Public Health Service Publication No. 1010, 1963.

Wade, Leo, et al., "Are Periodic Health Examinations Worthwhile?" *Annals of Internal Medicine*, Vol. 56, No. 1 (1964).

Utilization

Anderson, Odin W., "The Utilization of Health Services," in *Handbook of Medical Sociology*, edited by Howard E. Freeman, et al. Englewood Cliffs, N.J.: Prentice-Hall, Inc., 1963.

Blackwell, Barbara, "Anticipated Premedical Care Activities of Upper Middle Class Adults and Their Implications for Health Education Practice," *Health Education Monographs*, No. 17 (1964).

Byrne, Earl B.; William Schaffner; Eugene F. Dini; and George E. Case, "Infant Immunization Surveillance: Cost vs. Effect," *Journal of the American Medical Association*, Vol. 212, No. 5 (1970).

Coe, Rodney M., and Albert F. Wessen, "Social-Psychological Factors Influencing the Use of Community Health Services," *American Journal of Public Health*, Vol. 55, No. 7 (1965).

Freidson, Eliot, "The Organization of Medical Practice and Patient Behavior," *American Journal of Public Health*, Vol. 51, No. 1 (1961).

Goldsen, Rose K., "Patient Delay in Seeking Cancer Diagnosis: Behavioral Aspects," *Journal of Chronic Disease*, Vol. 16, No. 5 (1963).

Gordon, Gerald A., *Role Theory and Illness: A Sociological Perspective*. New Haven, Conn.: College and University Press, 1966.

Gray, Robert M., et al., "The Effects of Social Class and Friends' Expectations on Oral Polio Vaccination Participation," *American Journal of Public Health*, Vol. 56, No. 12 (1966).

Leventhal, Howard, "Fear Communications in the Acceptance of Preventive Health Practices," *Bulletin of New York Academy of Medicine*, Vol. 41, No. 11 (1965).

Leventhal, Howard, and Patricia N. Kafes, "The Effectiveness of Fear-Arousing Movies in Motivating Preventive Health Measures," *New York State Journal of Medicine*, Vol. 63, No. 6 (1963).

Kegeles, S.S., "Some Motives for Seeking Preventive Dental Care," *Journal of American Dental Association*, Vol. 67, No. 1 (1963).

MacDonald, Mary E., et al., "Special Factors in Relation to Participation in Follow-up Care of Rheumatic Fever," *Journal of Pediatrics*, Vol. 62, No. 4 (1963).

MacQueen, Ian A.G., "Can Health Education Ease the Load on Hospitals?" *Hospital World*, Vol. 3 (October 1964).

Mechanic, David, "The Sociology of Medicine: Viewpoints and Perspectives," *Journal of Health and Human Behavior*, Vol. 7, No. 4 (1966).

_____ , "The Concept of Illness Behavior," *Journal of Chronic Disease*, Vol. 15, No. 2 (1962).

Mechanic, David, and E.N. Volkart, "Stress, Illness Behavior, and the Sick Role," *American Sociological Review*, Vol. 26, No. 1 (1961).

Morris, Naomi M., et al., "Alienation as a Deterrent to Well-Child Supervision," *American Journal of Public Health*, Vol. 56, No. 11 (1966).

Ossenberg, Richard J., "The Experience of Deviance in the Patient Role: A Study of Class Differences," *Journal of Health and Human Behavior*, Vol. 3, No. 4 (1962).

Phillips, Derek L., "Self-Reliance and the Inclination to Adopt the Sick Role," *Social Forces*, Vol. 43, No. 4 (1965).

Reed, Elizabeth, "Education in an Oral Polio Vaccine Program," *Public Health Reports*, Vol. 78, No. 4 (1963).

Robbins, Paul R., "Some Explorations Into the Nature of Anxieties Relating to Illness," *Genetic Psychology Monographs*, Vol. 66 (1962).

Russell, Robert D., and Paul R. Robbins, "Health Education and the Use of Fear: A New Look," *Journal of School Health*, Vol. 34, No. 6 (1964).

Schulman, Sam and Anne Smith, "The Concept of Health Among Spanish-Speaking Villagers of New Mexico and Colorado," *Journal of Health and Human Behavior*, Vol. 4, No. 4 (1963).

Stoeckle, John D., et al., "On Going to See the Doctor, The Contributions of the Patient to the Decision to Seek Medical Care," *Journal of Chronic Disease*, Vol. 16, No. 9 (1963).

Patient Compliance

Berkowitz, Norman H., et al., "Patient Follow-through in an Outpatient Department," *Nursing Research*, Vol. 12, No. 1 (1963).

Berry, David, et al., "Self-Medication Behavior as Measured by Urine Chemical Tests in Domicillary Tuberculous Patients," *American Review of Respiratory Disease*, Vol. 86, No. 1 (1962).

Curtis, Elizabeth B., "Medication Errors Made by Patients," *Nursing Outlook*, Vol. 9, No. 5 (1961).

Davis, Milton S., "Variations in Patients' Compliance with Doctors' Orders: Analysis of Congruence Between Survey Responses and Results of Empirical Investigations," *Journal of Medical Education*, Vol. 41, No. 11, Pt. 1 (1966).

Davis, Milton S., and Robert L. Eichhorn, "Compliance with Medical Regimens: A Panel Study," *Journal of Health and Human Behavior*, Vol. 4, No. 4 (1963).

Hochstrasser, Donald, and Sally Lerner, "Behavioral Factors Affecting Medical Supervision of Nonhospitalized Tuberculosis Patients," *American Review of Respiratory Disease*, Vol. 91, No. 5 (1965).

Johannsen, W.J., et al., "On Accepting Medical Recommendations—Experiences with Patients in a Cardiac Work Classification Unit," *Archives of Environmental Health*, Vol. 12, No. 1 (1966).

Pragoff, Hale, "Adjustment of Tuberculosis Patients One Year After Hospital Discharge," *Public Health Reports*, Vol. 77, No. 8 (1962).

Preston, D.F., and F.L. Miller, "The Tuberculous Outpatient's Defection from Therapy," *American Journal of Medical Science*, Vol. 247, No. 1 (1964).

Schwartz, Doris, et al., "Medication Errors Made by Elderly Chronically Ill Patients," *American Journal of Public Health*, Vol. 52, No. 12 (1962).

Veracaris, Constantine A., "Social Factors Associated With the Acceptance of Medical Innovations: A Pilot Study," *Journal of Health and Human Behavior*, Vol. 3, No. 3 (1962).

Self-Care Programs

Allan, Frank N., "Current Concepts in Therapy: Education of the Diabetic Patient," *New England Journal of Medicine*, Vol. 268, No. 2 (1963).

Beckscheider, Joan, "The Use of Self as the Essence of Clinical Supervision in Ambulatory Patient Care," *Nursing Clinics of North America*, Vol. 6, No. 4 (1971).

Egbert, Lawrence D., et al., "Reduction of Postoperative Pain by Encouragement and Instruction of Patients," *New England Journal of Medicine*, Vol. 270, No. 16 (1964).

Ellis, Edward V., "Patient Education for Diabetics," *Health Education at Work*, Vol. 16 (1965).

Gates, Edwin W., "Diabetic Patient Education Clinic," *Today's Hospital* (March 1965).

Hallburg, Jeanne C., "Teaching Patients Self-Care," *Nursing Clinics of North America*, Vol. 5, No. 2 (1970).

James, Vernon L., and Warren E. Wheeler, "The Care-by-Patient Unit," *Pediatrics*, Vol. 43, No. 4 (1964).

Merrill, J.P.; E. Schupak; E. Cameron; and C.L. Hampers, "Hemodialysis in the Home," *Journal of the American Medical Association*, Vol. 190, No. 468 (1964).

O'Neill, Mary, "Guidelines for Teaching Home Dialysis," *Nursing Clinics of North America*, Vol. 6, No. 4 (1971).

Rosenberg, Stanley G., "Patient Education Leads to Better Care for Heart Patients," *HSMHA Technical Reports*, Vol. 86, No. 9 (1971).

Slowie, Linda A., "Patient Learning—Segments from Case Histories," *Journal of the American Dietetic Association*, Vol. 59 (1971).

Williams, Barbara Paul, "The Burned Patient's Need for Teaching," *Nursing Clinics of North America*, Vol. 6, No. 4 (1971).

Patient Beliefs and Attitudes

American Cancer Society, "New Study for the A.C.S. Shows Public Attitudes Toward Cancer Tests and Checkups," *Cancer News*, Vol. 20, No. 2 (1966).

Baumann, Barbara, "Diversities in Conceptions of Health and Physical Fitness," *Journal of Health and Human Behavior*, Vol. 2, No. 1 (1961).

Beasley, Joseph D., et al., "Attitudes and Knowledge Relevant to Family Planning Among New Orleans Negro Women," *American Journal of Public Health*, Vol. 56, No. 11 (1966).

Brooke, Melvin S., et al., "Reaction of Mothers to Literature on Child Rearing," *American Journal of Public Health*, Vol. 54, No. 5 (1964).

Freidson, Eliot, *Patients' Views of Medical Practice*. New York: Russell Sage Foundation, 1961.

Fulghum, J.E., and R.J. Klein, "Community Cancer Demonstration Project in Dade County, Florida," *Public Health Reports*, Vol. 77, No. 2 (1962).

Hartley, Eugene L., "Determinants of Health Beliefs and Behavior: 1. Psychological Determinants," *American Journal of Public Health*, Vol. 51, No. 10 (1961).

Horn, Daniel, and Selwyn Waingrow, "What Changes Are Occurring in Public Opinion Toward Cancer: National Public Opinion Survey," *American Journal of Public Health*, Vol. 54, No. 3 (1964).

Jenkins, C.D., "Group Differences in Perception: A Study of Community Beliefs and Feelings about Tuberculosis," *American Journal of Sociol.*, Vol. 71, No. 4 (1966).

_____, "The Semantic Differential for Health: A Technique for Measuring Beliefs about Diseases," *Public Health Reports*, Vol. 81, No. 6 (1966).

Kegeles, S.S., et al., "Survey of Beliefs About Cancer Detection and Taking Papanicolaou Tests," *Public Health Reports*, Vol. 80, No. 9 (1965).

Kirscht, John P., et al., "A National Study of Health Reliefs," *Journal of Health and Human Behavior*, Vol. 7, No. 4 (1966).

Miyaska, Tado and K. Fujii, "Knowledge and Attitudes of Housewives on Cancer," *Bulletin of the Institute of Public Health*, Vol. 14, No. 3 (1965).

Health Education Practices:
Learning and Teaching

Bharara, Sardool S., "For the Eradication of Smallpox: Joining Science and Tradition," *International Journal of Health Education*, Vol. 9, No. 12 (1961).

Bruner, Jerome S., *Toward A Theory of Instruction*. Cambridge, Mass.: Belknap Press of Harvard University Press, 1966.

Callan, Laurence B., "Adapting the Windshield Survey Model to Community Health Education," *HSMHA Health Reports*, Vol. 86, No. 3 (1971).

Cornely, Paul B., and Stanley K. Bigman, *Cultural Considerations in Changing Health Attitudes* (3 volumes). Washington, D.C.: Howard University, December 1961.

Creighton, Helen, and Sister Gabrielle, "Group Teaching in Cajun Country," *Nursing Outlook*, Vol. 9, No. 12 (1961).

Cross, Joanne, and Carol R. Parsons, "Nurse-Teaching and Goal Directed Nurse-Teaching to Motivate Change in Food Selection Behavior in Hospitalized Patients," *Nursing Research*, Vol. 20, No. 5 (1971).

Elliott, Florence C., "Classes for People with Heart Disease," *Nursing Outlook*, Vol. 9, No. 3 (1961).

Erchov, V.S., "The Effectiveness of Posters—Results of Five Years of Research," *Journal of Health Education*, Vol. 6, No. 1 (1963).

Feldman, Jacob J., *The Dissemination of Health Information: A Case Study in Adult Learning*. Chicago: Aldine Publishing Co., 1966.

Garcia, Carmen S., "Evaluative Study of T-Group Experiences as a Teaching Method," in *Public Health Research in Puerto Rico*. Office of Research, School of Public Health, Puerto Rico, May 1965.

Glaser, Robert, "Learning and the Technology of Instruction," *Audio-Visual Communication Review*, Vol. 9, No. 5 (1961).

Green, Joan L., "Teaching the Patient with Hyocardial Infection," *Hospital Progress*, Vol. 42, No. 6 (1961).

Green, Morris and Mary Ann Durocher, "Improving Parent Care for Handicapped Children," *Children*, Vol. 12, No. 5 (September/October, 1965).

Hangartner, Carl J., "The Educational Role of the Hospital," *Hospital Progress*, Vol. 46, No. 6 (1965).

Holder, Lee, and S. Subbiah, "The Informal Approach in Health Education Activities," *Adult Leadership*, Vol. 11, No. 2 (1962).

Kinsella, Cynthia, "Educational Television for a Hospital System," *American Journal of Nursing*, Vol. 64, No. 1 (1964).

Klein, David, "Who Reads All These Pamphlets?" *Rehabilitation Literature*, Vol. 24, No. 6 (1963).

Krumboltz, J.D., "Evaluation of Programmed Instruction," in *Programmed Instruction in Medical Education*, edited by J.P. Lysaught. Rochester Clearinghouse, University of Rochester, New York, 1965.

Krysan, Germaine S., "How Do We Teach Four Million Diabetics?" *American Journal of Nursing*, Vol. 65, No. 11 (1965).

Lanese, Richard R., and Randolph S. Thrush, "Measuring Readability of Health Education Literature," *Journal of the American Dietetic Association*, Vol. 42, No. 3 (1963).

Leeds, William G., "A System of Diabetic Patient Instruction in a General Hospital," *Connecticut Medicine*, Vol. 25, No. 5 (1962).

Ley, Phillip, "Primacy, Rated Importance, and the Recall of Medical Statements," *Journal of Health and Social Behavior*, Vol. 13 (1972).

McCloy, James, "Production of Medical Programmers on Television," *Health Education Journal*, Vol. 19, No. 2 (1961).

McCormick, John G., and Leon J. Taubenhaus, "The Brookline Aging Project—Some Implications for Health Education," *Health Education Monographs*, No. 15 (1963).

McDonald, Glen W., and Mildred B. Kaufman, "Teaching Machines for Patients with Diabetes," *Journal of the American Dietetic Association*, Vol. 42, No. 3 (1963).

Meadows, Dorothy, "Patients Learn About Diabetes from Teaching Machines," *Hospitals*, Vol. 39, No. 24 (1965).

Medical Economics, Inc., "Printed Aids for Patients: Make the Most of Them," in *Doctor's Aide Program*, 1972.

Mohammed, Mary F.B., "Patients' Understanding of Written Health Information," *Nursing Research*, Vol. 13, No. 2 (1964).

Nickerson, Hiram, "A Teaching Machine for Diabetic Patients—A Study Report," *Journal of the Maine Medical Association*, Vol. 54, No. 11 (1963).

Owen, John S., "Poster Evaluation," *Health Education Journal*, Vol. 20, No. 4 (1962).

Painton, J. Frederick, "Education of the Diabetic Patient," *Bulletin of the Millard Fillmore Hospital*, Buffalo, New York, Vol. 11 (1964).

Palm, Mary Lock, "Recognizing Opportunities for Informal Patient Teaching," *Nursing Clinics of North America*, Vol. 6, No. 4 (1971).

Pender, Janice L., "Dietitian Teaches Patients Via Closed-Circuit TV," *Hospital Topics*, Vol. 44, No. 2 (1966).

Reinstein, Norbert, "Educational Implications of the Madison Study," *The Crusader*, Wisconsin Anti-TB Association, Vol. 57, No. 4 (1964).

Roberts, Beryl J., et al., "An Experimental Study of Two Approaches to Communication," *American Journal of Public Health*, Vol. 53, No. 9 (1963).

Robinson, Geraldine, and Marilyn Filkins, "Group Teaching with Out-patients," *American Journal of Nursing*, Vol. 64, No. 11 (1964).

Scott, John F., and Howard E. Freeman, "The One Night Stand in Mental Health Education," *Social Problems*, Vol. 10, No. 3 (1963).

Shapiro, L.R., et al., "Dietary Survey for Planning a Local Nutrition Program," *Public Health Reports*, Vol. 77, No. 3 (1962).

Skiff, Anna, "Programmed Instruction and Patient Teaching," *American Journal of Public Health*, Vol. 55, No. 3 (1965).

Southworth, Warren H., "A Tuberculosis Survey: Findings and Implications," *International Journal of Health Education*, Vol. 8, No. 1 (1965).

Spiegel, Allen D., "Educating Patients, Having Patience, and Testing New Approaches," *Resident Physician*, Vol. 10, No. 9 (1964).

_____ , "Teaching Diabetic Patients Through Automation," *Hospital Topics*, Vol. 42, No. 8 (1964).

Spiegel, Allen D., and George S. Buis, "TV Brings the Classroom to the Patients," *Modern Hospital*, Vol. 100, No. 2 (1963).

Thrush, Randolph S., and Richard R. Lanese, "The Use of Printed Material in Diabetes Education," *Diabetes*, Vol. 2, No. 2 (1962).

Torribrio, J.A., and L.H. Glass, "Venereal Disease Exhibit at Teenage Fair," *Public Health Reports*, Vol. 80, No. 1 (1965).

Varvara, Filomena F., "Teaching the Patient About Open Heart Surgery," *American Journal of Nursing*, Vol. 65, No. 10 (1965).

Vavra, Catherine E., et al., "Meeting the Challenge of Educational Care in Heart Disease," *American Journal of Public Health*, Vol. 56, No. 9 (1966).

Weaver, Barbara, and Elsie L. Williams, "Teaching the Tuberculosis Patient," *American Journal of Nursing*, Vol. 63, No. 12 (1963).

Whealy, Elizabeth, and F.R. Wake, "Pamphlets and Changes in Behavior: Experimental Evidence," *Canadian Journal of Public Health*, Vol. 54, No. 2 (1963).

Young, Marjorie A.C., "Review of Research Related to Health Education Communications: Methods and Materials," *Health Education Monographs*, No. 25 (1967).

Zachert, Virginia, and P.L. Wilde, "Student Attitudes Toward a Programmed Course," *Journal of Medical Education*, Vol. 39, No. 9 (1964).

5

A Review of Productivity in Dentistry

Paul J. Feldstein*

Introduction

This chapter deals with manpower productivity in dental care. We first discuss elements of the supply of dental care, and then examine the potential for increased productivity by use of auxiliary personnel; in the process, the literature on dental manpower productivity is reviewed. The rest of the chapter deals with restraints on the use of auxiliaries, needed research, and policy implications.

Background: The Supply of Dental Care

The Stock of Dentists

There are approximately 120,000 dentists in the United States, or 1,685 persons per dentist.[1] The number of active dentists are estimated to be approximately 104,000 or a population-dentist ratio of 1967:1. The number of active dentists has increased 33 percent between 1950 and 1970, or 1.44 percent per year.

Changes in the stock of dentists could occur as a result of deaths and retirements or by additions as a result of the production of new graduates and by the immigration of foreign trained dentists. In 1970, 373 foreign dentists immigrated to the U.S. However, except for Canadian trained dentists, licensing boards do not permit foreign trained dentists to practice unless they have undergone additional training. It is thus not possible to determine how many of the foreign trained dentists were Canadian or how many actually completed their additional training and were permitted to practice. Increments to the stock of U.S. dentists by foreign trained dentists are thus likely to be small.

There were 53 dental schools in the U.S. in 1970 and these produced 3,500 dental graduates in that year. It is estimated that by 1975 there will be 57 dental schools with an annual production of 4,270 graduates. The major determinant of additions to the stock of dentists therefore is the number of dental schools and their number of spaces. The demand for spaces by prospective students has continually exceeded the available spaces and in recent years the percent of

*Professor of Economics, University of Michigan.

applicants enrolled has dropped to 42 percent (1969-1970). Thus the constraint on increases in the stock of dentists is the requirement—in addition to examination and licensing—of having taken a dental education in an approved school, with minimum educational requirements. Since the annual increase in dental graduates has been 1.76 percent (1955-1970), any further increases in the output of dental care would have to come from increases in the productivity of existing dentists.

The Production of Dental Services

More than 75 percent of dentists are nonsalaried and in solo practice. Although the percent of dentists that are specialists are increasing (3.1 percent in 1955 and 8.5 percent in 1969), more than 85 percent of the practicing dentists are still general practitioners. The predominant form of reimbursement is fee-for-service.

For purposes of analyzing the dental sector it is useful to view the dentist as a "firm" producing dental services. The factor inputs, broadly defined, include the dentist's own time, the time of any auxiliary personnel, equipment such as number of chairs and type of drill, as well as office expenses and dental supplies. In the production of dental services, the dentist must work within a framework of technology which constrains his possible choices of combinations of factor inputs. "Technology," broadly defined, can be taken to cover the methods known to the dentist, the type of equipment available, and the duties which his assistants are allowed to perform. In the short run (the time in which the number of dentists are fixed) increased output of dental services can come from reorganization of the methods of dental practice or from increased productivity of the individual dental practices. To date, there is little, if any, information on the effect of different methods of dental practice on dental output.

The main cause of past increases in dental productivity, and the likely source of future increases, lies in increased use of dental auxiliaries. Dentist hours worked have decreased, and therefore increased production can most rapidly occur by hiring more auxiliaries to do "standard" auxiliary functions and/or by delegating tasks traditionally performed by the dentist to the auxiliaries. This chapter will concentrate on these labor intensive approaches toward increasing productivity.[2]

Increased Dental Productivity from Increased Use of Auxiliaries

Past Trends in Dental Productivity

Several measures of output have been used to describe the increase in dental productivity: dental visits, consumer expenditures on dental care, and gross income of dentists.

When visits are used as the measure of output, the increase in productivity (visits per dentist) from 1950 to 1970 has been 1.6 percent per year. (When a shorter period is used 1955 to 1970, the annual percent increase is lower, 1.2 percent.) Over the same time period, the number of auxiliaries has increased from 1.04 to 1.40 per dentist, or an increase of 1.5 percent per year (1.1 percent per year from 1955). The annual increase in dental productivity and in use of auxiliaries appears to be closely related. A more accurate indication of the contribution of auxiliaries to the increased number of dental visits is shown in Table 5-1. This shows, for each of three years for which data is available, the number of visits per dentist with different numbers of dental auxiliaries. According to this table, with increased use of auxiliaries, a dentist can increase his output by 20 to 40 percent.

When consumer expenditures on dental care (adjusted by the dental care price index) are used as the measure of dental output, then from 1950 to 1970 the annual increase in dental productivity has been 3.1 percent. The larger annual percent increase in dental productivity, when deflated consumer expenditures on dental care are used as the measure of dental output, may result from the fact that the average dental visit has changed over time, and that this change is incorporated in the expenditure data but not the visit data.

The third measure of dental output that may be used is gross incomes of dentists. If dentists employed different numbers of auxiliaries and the price of dental care was similar among the dentists, then differences in their gross incomes would represent differences in output. For each of the years analyzed, gross incomes per dentist increased with increased numbers of auxiliaries. In

Table 5-1

Average Annual Patient Visits per Dentist by Number of Auxiliary Personnel Employed

Year[a]	Auxiliaries Employed (Full-Time Personnel Only)[f]				
	0	1	2	3	4 or more
1958[c]	2272	3014	3174	3929	b
1961[d]	2003	2968	3706	4790	b
1964[e]	2355	3015	3946	4409	6170

[a]Data incomplete, unavailable, or unreliable for 1950, 1953, 1956, and 1968, *Surveys of Dental Practice.*

[b]Too few Survey replies for reliable statistics.

[c]Source: American Dental Association, *The 1959 Survey of Dental Practice*, p. 47.

[d]Source: American Dental Association, *The 1962 Survey of Dental Practice*, p. 45.

[e]Source: American Dental Association, *The 1965 Survey of Dental Practice*, p. 35.

[f]Auxiliaries include dental technicians, dental hygienists, dental assistants, and secretaries/receptionists.

more recent years, however, the increases in gross income for each dentist-auxiliary combination have been lower.

When gross income per dentist was used to measure the increased productivity over time, it was found that gross income per dentist per hour (adjusted for dental price increases) increased 3.1 percent annually from 1955 to 1970.

Regardless of whether the output measure is visits, expenditures on dental care or gross incomes of dentists, it is apparent that dentists could achieve substantial increases in productivity (1.6 to 3.1 percent per year) by employing additional auxiliary personnel.[3]

*Potential Increase in Productivity by Use
of Expanded Function Auxiliaries*

There is mounting evidence that the use of "expanded function auxiliaries" (EFAs) can lead to appreciable increases in dental productivity. In several foreign countries, notably New Zealand, EFAs are being effectively utilized on a large scale. The general conclusions to be drawn from this evidence and foreign experiences are: (1) auxiliaries can be trained, in a relatively short time, to perform many functions traditionally performed by the dentist, at the same level of quality provided by the dentist; and (2) the output of dental services provided by the dentist can be increased through the employment of EFAs.[4]

In a study conducted in Louisville, Kentucky (Lotzkar et al., 1967) by the Division of Mental Health, dental assistants received 48 weeks training to perform additional tasks. Using a "procedures completed per day" measure of output, a team of one dentist and four EFAs was 133 percent more productive than a "traditional" team of one dentist, one chairside assistant, and other "office" help. Using a "time unit" measure of work, the EFA team increased productivity by 133 percent over the "traditional" team. A team of one dentist and *three* EFAs treated 62 percent more patients, performed 84 percent more procedures, and accomplished 80 percent more time units than did the "traditional" team. The work performed by the EFAs was highly satisfactory from a professional viewpoint, and the patients treated indicated a high degree of satisfaction with the work provided.

A continuing study conducted by the University of Alabama (Hammons, 1967, 1968, and 1971) involved the delegation of expanded functions to "dental therapists," high school graduates who were given two years training in the performance of various intraoral tasks. The therapists were found to perform as well as dentists in inserting and finishing amalgam and silicate restorations, inserting temporary fillings, and placing matrix bands for amalgam restorations. In fact, the quality of work done by the therapists was often found to be better than that rendered by advanced dental students.

In a study conducted by the Department of Indian Health (Abramowitz,

1965), dental health teams consisting of one dentist and two assistants were organized. The assistants were Indian women who received eight weeks training, including one week on "clinic management." The assistants selected, contoured, placed, and removed matrix bands, placed alloys, and served Class II restorations; and the quality of their work was comparable to that of dentists.

A program conducted by the Philadelphia Department of Public Health (Soricelli, 1971) utilized "technotherapists," former dental assistants who received six months additional training. The technotherapists then performed many technical services traditionally handled by dentists, including virtually everything in the area of operative dentistry except the injection of local anesthetic, the cutting of cavity preparations, and certain other functions. The work of the technotherapists was found to be highly satisfactory in comparison to that done by dentists, and even the quality of work performed by the dentists themselves was found to be upgraded, due perhaps to the "competition" provided by the technotherapists. Teams of one dentist, three technotherapists, two assistants, and one clerk were found to be capable of doing as much work as four dentists each working with one chairside assistant. This productivity increase is an overstatement in that the functions performed extended only to examinations, cleanings, and fillings; but it is an understatement in that the teams were forced to use a facility not well-suited to efficient operation of the team.

In an experiment conducted at Great Lakes Naval Training Center (Ludwig, 1963 and 1964), dental "technicians" received 23 weeks training on dental anatomy, dental materials, oral hygiene, applying rubberdams, inserting cavity liners or bases, placing matrix bands, and inserting and finishing amalgam and silicate fillings. The quality of work done by the technicians in performing these functions was deemed to be "as satisfactory as conventional methods." The combination of one dentist and four technicians, working at three chairs, was found to be highly efficient. Some dentists increased productivity by over 80 percent, and treated twice as many patients, using this setup as compared to the conventional "one-chair" operation.

A program conducted in the Canadian military (Baird et al., 1962) took experienced "clinical technicians" (the counterparts of civilian dental hygienists) and gave them four weeks training on an *individualized* basis in expanded functions. The training was in functions similar to those performed by the "technicians" in the Great Lakes study, plus training in certain simple standard procedures in prosthodontics and periodontics. When the technician was added to a "team" of one dentist, one chairside assistant, and one roving assistant, team productivity increased 99.1 percent, of which 61.7 percent was attributed directly to the technician's participation and 37.4 percent to increased productivity by the other members of the team. Other teams, composed of one dentist and one technician, accomplished on the average in a 6.5 hour day the same amount of work done by a dentist working alone in 10.5 hours—a 61.5 percent increase. (Three treatment rooms were necessary to effectively utilize these "two-man" teams.) Further, the dentists involved were able to make more productive use of their time due to the technicians' participation. The percent of his time which the average dentist spent actually operating increased from 49.8 percent to 75.0 percent; and the dentist spent less time idle or doing "nonproductive" work such as greeting patients, etc.

In several foreign countries, dental care providers, faced with a shortage of dental manpower, have turned to expanded function auxiliaries with successful results. The leading example is the New England dental nurse program (Walsh, 1965). The nurses are trained to provide initial examination and charting, prophylaxis, topical application of fluorides, operative dentistry for deciduous and permanent teeth, extraction of teeth, and dental health education. When trained, each nurse becomes responsible for the dental health care of approximately 500 school children. Groups of 80 nurses are monitored and supervised by one dentist. Surveys indicate that the program has resulted in better oral health for patients, and that the work done by the nurses has been of high quality. Use of this system has made possible the provision of a much greater supply of dental care to the people of New Zealand than would otherwise be available, given their supply of dentists.

A survey conducted by Leatherman (1968) found that "there has been a marked increase in the training and use of the New Zealand-type nurses in the developing countries and Australia." In 1960, six countries were using New Zealand-type nurses in public dental services, while by 1968, fourteen countries were utilizing this auxiliary. The nurses are typically trained for two years, and perform intraoral functions including regular examination, prophylaxis, filling of teeth, extraction of teeth under local anesthesia, and radiographic examination. Leatherman forecasts that, in the future, these nurses will be allowed to work with less and less direct supervision by a dentist. Leatherman also predicted more and more delegation of comprehensive duties to dental *hygienists*.

Arnold (1969) has concluded that the delegation of certain functions to a properly trained clinical chairside assistant would save fifty percent of the dentists' time normally needed for a filling. These functions include taking impressions for study costs, placing and removing rubberdama and matrix bands, condensing and carving amalgam restorations in previously-prepared teeth, placing of silicate and acrylic restorations in previously-prepared teeth, applying the final finish and polish to the above-listed restorations, and placing and removing temporary restorations. The World Health Organization (1969) has advised nations with dental health programs to expand their dental services by the utilization of auxiliary personnel (including chairside assistants, laboratory technicians, hygienists, and EFAs) and the development of dental health teams.

It is thus apparent that the dental "firm" can increase its output of services by greater use of auxiliary personnel, especially through the delegation to auxiliaries of tasks traditionally performed by the dentist. Most of the demonstrations in this country and the foreign experiences with EFAs support the finding of more services per dentist through greater use of dental auxiliaries. The dentist is thus freed for other, more complicated tasks, and the total amount of services produced per dentist is increased, with no reduction in quality of care.

To date, however, certain restraints have prevented the full utilization of EFAs in this country.

Restraints on the Full Use of Auxiliary Personnel

Dental Practice Acts

The dental practice acts in all states have for a long time constituted a severe restraint on the delegation of expanded functions to auxiliaries. This is particularly true with respect to dental hygienists. The typical, traditional statute (*Michigan Compiled Laws Annotated* § 338.209) defines the functions of hygienists as follows:

Such licensed hygienists may remove calcerous deposits, accretions, and stains from the teeth, and may prescribe or apply ordinary mouthwashes of soothing character, but shall not perform any other operation on the teeth, mouth, or tissues of the oral cavity, or administer any therapeutic remedies to diseased portions of teeth or their surrounding tissues.

The hygienist is thus legally allowed to perform only functions which are far less complex than those for which she has been trained. Delegation of functions is further inhibited by the legal requirement in virtually all states, that any work performed by the hygienist be done under the "direct supervision" of the dentist. Such dental practice acts therefore limit the use of auxiliary personnel, and so constitute a limitation on potential increases in output.

State Dental Examining Boards

State dental examining (licensing) boards apparently have substantial powers to define the functions of auxiliaries. This is particularly true with respect to assistants, whose functions are typically not defined in the statutes themselves.[5] To the extent that the definition of auxiliary functions becomes a matter of discretionary power of state boards, rather than of inflexible statutory requirements, greater delegation of functions to auxiliaries should be possible. However, since many licensing boards are composed of older practitioners, and are thus more conservative,[6] the "liberalizing" effect of this change may not be very great. Johnson and Bernstein (1972) concluded that, despite revised dental practice sets in almost half the states, "It appears that very few additional functions have been delegated to dental hygienists commensurate with their level of training. . . . It appears dental assistants are still not allowed to do a considerable number of functions that they should be able to perform in line with their experience and education."

Practitioner Attitudes

The attitudes of dental practitioners also constitute a barrier to the use of EFAs. One survey of practitioners (Brown, 1967) concluded that many dentists are reluctant to assign technical tasks to auxiliaries because they feel technical competence to be the most important trademark of a fine practitioner. The surveyed dentists also disliked having to perform supervisory functions or to teach new personnel, and felt that it was necessary to deal with patients personally in order to maintain good "dentist-patient" relationships. Hall's study found similar negative attitudes toward auxiliaries among Canadian dentists.

It appears, however, that younger practitioners have more liberal attitudes toward the utilization of auxiliaries. The Brown study found that younger practitioners and recent graduates are more likely to delegate tasks to assistants than are older practitioners.

Suggested Research

Although it would appear that the measurement of output in the dental sector is less complicated than the measurement of output in the medical care sector, it is still not without its problems. Future studies of dental productivity should examine the different output mixes that are produced when different combinations of dentists and auxiliaries are used. Instead of productivity gains, the use of more auxiliaries might result in a greater number of visits that are performed primarily by auxiliaries. The output (visit) mix might thus be different than when a greater proportion of the dentists input is used.

Further research on dental productivity should also seek to determine more precisely the contribution to dental output of each type of dental auxiliary and of different numbers of such auxiliaries. Estimates of the effect on dental productivity of the nonlabor inputs and technical change are also needed. With regard to expanded function auxiliaries, what further tasks, now handled by the dentist, can auxiliaries perform and at what level of training? And finally, how can practitioner attitudes on the use of auxiliaries, especially expanded function auxiliaries, be changed?

Notes

1. The data on the supply of dental services are based upon Paul J. Feldstein (1973).

2. Maurizi (1969) attempted to measure the annual percent increase in dentist productivity attributable to technical change over time. He compared the change in dentist time-input required to perform various types of services between 1943 and 1950 and between 1943 and 1958. The result of his calculations were that technical change increased output by approximately one percent per year between 1943 and 1950. Using some of the earlier data, Maurizi adjusted the dentist time-input by age of dentists and derived a second estimate of increased output due to technical change of 0.84 per year.

(Maurizi also estimated a production function based upon cross-section data from the 1961 *Survey of Dental Practice.* The estimated function is:

$$\log VPD = 0.62798 + 0.466 \log AUX + 0.77 \log HRD + 0.254 \log CHR$$

where *VPD* = annual patient visits per dentist; *AUX* = number of auxiliary personnel employed by the dentist; *HRD* = annual hours worked by the dentist; and *CHR* = number of chairs in the office.)

Another study by the American Council on Education (1961), estimated the time saved, hence additional cavities filled and bridges placed, of using high-speed cutting equipment. "The total theoretical saving of dentists' time from the use of high speed equipment is, therefore, the equivalent of 1,741 dentists (over the period 1950 to 1975)" (p. 478). Assuming (among other things) that the number of dentists in 1975 were to be 115,000, then this savings in time would represent a 1.5 average annual increase in dentist productivity.

These findings must be considered highly tentative due to data limitations, but they suggest an annual productivity increase due to technological change of about one percent.

3. Studies of dental practices in Canada have yielded similar results. Hall (1965) found that Canadian dentists who use assistants see more patients per day. Those dentists surveyed who employed no assistants averaged 10 to 12 patients per day; dentists with one full-time assistant averaged 15 to 17 patients per day; and dentists using two to four full-time assistants saw 16 to 20 patients per day. Although Hall did not collect gross income data, he did find that those dentists with higher *net* income tended to make greater use of auxiliaries than did those dentists who earned less.

4. For a summary of the literature in this area see D.B. Ast (1972).

5. The Minnesota dental practices act expressly delegates rule-making authority to the licensing board: "(The) dentist shall permit such unlicensed assistant

to perform only those acts which he is authorized to delegate to unlicensed assistants by the board of dentistry. The board may permit differing levels of dental assistance upon recognized education standards, approved by the board, for the training of dental assistants." See *Minnesota Statutes Annotated* § 150A.10 (Sub. 2).

6. Some state dental practice acts expressly exclude members of dental school faculties from eligibility for membership on the state examining board.

Bibliography

Abramowitz, Joseph, "Expanded Functions for Dental Assistants: A Preliminary Study," *Journal of the American Dental Association*, Vol. 72: 386 (February 1965).

American Council on Education, *The Survey of Dentistry*. Washington, D.C.: American Council on Education, 1961.

Arnold., G., "The Dental Assistant, the Clinical Chairside Assistant and the Dental Hygienist as Members of the Dental Team in General Practice," *International Dental Journal*, Vol. 19: 12 (1969).

Ast, D.C., "Changes in Oral Health Delivery Systems Resulting from Implementation of More Efficient Preventive Measures and Greater Delegation of Responsibilities to Auxiliaries," *Oral Health, Dentistry and the American Public*, William Brown (ed.), Norman Okla.: University of Oklahoma Press, 1974.

Baird, K.M.; D.B. Shillington; and D.H. Protheroe, "Pilot Study on the Advanced Training and Employment of Auxiliary Dental Personnel in the Royal Canadian Dental Corps: Preliminary Report," *Canadian Dental Association Journal*, Vol. 28: 627 (October 1962).

Brown, William E., "Increasing Productivity and Reducing Disease. The Dental Health Team: Potential Role of Auxiliaries," *Journal of the American Dental Association*, Vol. 75: 882 (October 1967).

Feldstein, Paul J., *Financing Dental Care: An Economic Analysis*. Lexington, Mass.: Lexington Books, D.C. Heath, 1973.

Hall, Oswald, *Utilization of Dentists in Canada*. Royal Commission on Health Services, Ottowa, Canada: Queens Printer, 1965.

Hammons, P.E., and H.C. Jamison, "Expanded Functions for Dental Auxiliaries," *Journal of the American Dental Association*, Vol. 75: 658 (1967).

_____ , "Increasing the Production of Dental Auxiliaries," *Journal of the American College of Dentists*, Vol. 35: 154 (1968).

Hammons, P.E.; H.C. Jamison, and L.L. Wilson, "Quality of Services Provided by Dental Therapists in an Experimental Program at the University of Alabama," *Journal of the American Dental Association*, Vol. 82: 1060 (1971).

Johnson, D.W., and S. Bernstein, "Classification of States Regarding Expanding Duties for Dental Auxiliaries and Selected Aspects of Dental Licensure," *American Journal of Public Health*, Vol. 62: 208 (February 1972).

Leatherman, G.H., "Survey of Auxiliary Dental Personnel," *International Dental Journal*, Vol. 19: 49 (1968).

Lotzkar, S.; D.W. Johnson; and M.B. Thompson, "Experimental Program On Expanded Functions for Dental Assistants: Phase 3 Experiment with Dental Teams," *Journal of the American Dental Association*, Vol. 82 (1967).

Ludwig, W.E.; E.O. Schoebelen; and R.J. Knoedler, *Greater Utilization of Dental Technicians, I. Report of Training.* Great Lakes, Ill.: U.S. Naval Training Center, Dental Research Facility, 1963.

_____, *Greater Utilization of Dental Technicians, II. Report of Clinical Tests.* Great Lakes, Ill.: U.S. Naval Training Center, Dental Research Facility, 1964.

Maurizi, Alex, *Economic Essays on the Dental Profession.* College of Business Administration, University of Iowa, 1969.

Soricelli, D.A., "Practical Experience in Peer Review Controlling Quality in the Delivery of Dental Care," *American Journal of Public Health*, Vol. 61: 2046 (October 1971).

Walsh, John P., "The Dental Nurse," *American College of Dentists Journal*, Vol. 32: 62 (1965).

World Health Organization, *Report of the Expert Committee on Dental Auxiliary Personnel.* Geneva, Switzerland: WHO, Technical Report Series No. 163, 1969.

6

Occupational Licensure and Health Care Productivity: The Issues and the Literature

H.E. Frech*

Introduction

Key issues in health manpower policy revolve around occupational licensure. It forms an important part of the legal and regulatory framework within which medical care is produced, and it has a direct bearing on the training and use of health manpower. These, in turn, affect the productivity of the health services industry in the most basic sense. Even small changes in licensure conditions may be expected to dominate other policy changes.

This chapter will review the literature relating to the impact of licensure on productivity in the health sector, and relating to the policy issues which licensure raises. It draws not only on the writing of economists but on that of physicians, public health specialists, historians, lawyers, and others.

Analysis of the Origins of Licensure in General

In examination of the origin or causes of licensure, two closely-related studies have been undertaken—those by Moore (1961) and by Stigler (1971). In the Moore study, two models for the determination of the political strength of the licensure movement are proposed: one is based on protection of the public interest, and the other holds that licensure is designed to confer monopoly power on the members of the profession. Stigler uses similar models. Both studies use the year of licensure as a proxy for the strength of the licensure movement in various occupations. Stigler also examines some characteristics of currently licensed occupations. Their differing interpretations illustrate the basic controversy running through analyses of licensure.

Moore finds the earliness-of-licensure to be positively and statistically significantly related to the educational level of the occupation and its total income. He believes this to be consistent with the public interest theory because the public most needs protection in relatively complex occupations and in those which make up an important part of consumer budgets. Stigler, on the other hand, finds the same earliness-of-licensure measure to be positively and significantly

*Assistant Professor of Economics, University of California at Santa Barbara.

related to two proxies for the political power of an occupational group—relative size and extent of urbanization. Further, by comparing occupations currently licensed with those only licensed in some states and those nowhere licensed, he demonstrates that licensed occupations tend to be more stable in membership and to have higher incomes; both of these are again proxies for the political power of the occupation. Licensed occupations also tend to be self-employed occupations, so that concentrated employer political opposition to licensure is absent. And, occupations in national markets, where a state's licensure could be relatively easily avoided by the employers' movement to other states, tend not to be licensed. Stigler believes that this evidence is consistent with the theory that occupations seek licensure to further their interests.

Stigler's analysis of the characteristics of licensed occupations is, of course, beset with "simultaneous equation" bias: licensure doubtless *causes* some of the characteristics of licensed occupations. Stigler's ordinary least squares regressions overstate the importance of the occupational characteristics as determinants of licensure, to the extent that some causation runs from licensure to characteristics. This problem can be avoided by the use of simultaneous estimating methods. In any case, the facts about which professions tend to be licensed seems clear, while the interpretation of these facts is still open to discussion.

Licensure, Certification, and Information

In health, the idealistic or public interest theory of occupational licensure was invoked when licensure was originally sought. Licensure was said to protect the public from dishonest and incompetent practitioners, and it was to raise the standards for professional entry and provide valuable public assurance that each licensed person would possess the requisite skill and knowledge. This still stands as the predominant interpretation of both the purpose and effect of health licensure. An alternate notion, however, the acquired regulation theory, holds that the purpose of licensure was to restrict entry into the professions concerned, and to provide more professional control of the behavior of individual professionals (see Rottenberg, 1962).

It may be of some relevance that, in health, licensure was sought by the profession rather than by the public, though it was the latter which was to be protected.[1] Also, the medical profession's leadership appears to have been aware of the implications of licensure on physician supply. The head of the AMA's Council on Medical Education said (Bevan, 1928, p. 1176):

... with the reduction of the number of medical schools from 160 to eighty, there occurred a market reduction in the number of medical students and medical graduates. We had anticipated this and felt that this was a desirable thing. We had ... a great over-supply of mediocre practitioners.

Of course, these two theories are not entirely mutually exclusive. No one's motives can be assumed to be either entirely altruistic nor entirely selfish, and social science theories attempt only to explain observed behavior, not the motives of those concerned. The aim is to determine which theory provides the most useful illumination, not to argue that any simple theory explains everything. Further, it is quite possible that licensure, even if it is sought by the profession rather than by the public, may well benefit the public in any event.

In addition, there also exists a possible alternative to licensure—one which might provide just as much consumer information, and which would thus allow consumers to make informed choices among health workers. This alternative is certification, also called "permissive licensing." Under a certification system, practitioners would meet a standard in order to be certified, just as under licensing, but noncertified personnel would also be permitted to offer the service. Thus, a consumer would know that all certified individuals possess some minimal level of skills and knowledge necessary for certification. Many argue that if they still choose the less qualified provider, theirs is an informed choice. Further, varying levels of qualifications might be graded "A," "B," and so on, thus providing even better information than is provided by current licensure. Such a certification system could be either private or governmental.

The Issue of Medical Care Quality

A variant of the idealistic theory of occupational licensure holds that licensure was necessary because the quality of medical care was too low. One may interpret this kind of statement in two ways. If it means that consumers were *fooled*, in the absence of licensure, into purchasing lower quality services than they prefer, this merely restates the argument that licensure provides valuable information. It may be argued, of course, that certification can provide the same information, but without limiting consumer choice.

The alternate interpretation of this argument is that, even if consumers had perfect information, they would consume services of insufficient quality. This is a somewhat authoritarian position, quite different than that presented above, in that it prevents consumers from following their own values. However, while the imperfections in consumer knowledge suggest some credence in the view that consumers ought to be forced to consumer higher quality services than they might otherwise choose, it has not yet been clearly demonstrated that licensure regulation really does result in higher quality. Under licensing, by preventing entry of those with lower qualifications, the quality of care rendered *by licensed professionals* may rise, but consumer substitution of other services such as chiropractors, the advice of friends and self-treatment, plus provider substitution of lower-skilled personnel for expensive licensed individuals, could result in lower quality of care *actually received*. This kind of case has been forcefully made by a New Jersey health administrator (Stevens and Vermeulen, 1971, p. III-8):

It's easy to sit behind a desk in Chicago and frame ideals about the quality of care. But, a supposedly non-qualified doctor can put on a tourniquet and give the usual drugs and plasma for shock to tide the patient over until an American-trained doctor gets there. And that's better than having the patient die.

Results of Licensing in the Medical Care Market

The Licensing Mechanism

Licensure for American-trained physicians follows (1) attendance at a medical school approved by either the AMA or the American Association of Medical Colleges (the lists are identical) plus (2) service at an AMA-approved hospital internship program and (3) passage of a written examination. The test seems to be essentially a formality since about 94 percent of medical school graduates pass it.

Licensure for other types of health manpower follows a similar pattern, except that internship is usually not required, and the states are less uniform in their educational and examination requirements. In most cases, the relevant professional association is delegated much authority to determine requirements, especially for the accreditation of educational programs. (Licensure of foreign-trained professionals is quite different, and will be discussed below.)

Supply Restriction and Substitution

Restricting the supply of health professionals by licensing can of course be expected to directly raise the prices of their services. Conservative calculations presented by Sloan (1970, p. 49) indicate that the internal rate of return to medical education (four years of medical school plus one year of internship) in 1965 was 24.1 percent; by comparison, Becker (1964, p. 28) calculates returns of 13-15 percent for undergraduate college education. If one considers that the relevant investment opportunity for a college graduate would be 10 percent, the present value, at time of medical school admission, of the right to be admitted to medical school was $50,065, or roughly $5,200 per year (assuming a 35 year working life). Since median general practitioner income in 1965 was about $25,000 (Owens, 1970), this assumption of a 10 percent opportunity cost of capital would leave us with the estimate that licensure-caused medical school restrictions raised physician incomes by 25 percent. If we assume a 5 percent opportunity cost, the corresponding value of medical school admission is $127,224, which is approximately $7,800 per year, implying an increase in physician income of 45 percent.

The high cost of physicians time resulting from physicians' licensing causes some substitution of other inputs in the production of health. People may be more likely to substitute the advice of friends and self-treatment and to go to nonlicensed "quacks," faith healers, chiropractors, osteopaths, and other providers not subject to MD licensure. Those who do go to a physician may receive less attention from him. The physician may substitute more use of other individuals and machines (other inputs) for his time; to the extent that licensure laws prevent the physician from delegating more work to paramedical personnel, he has less time for each individual patient.

The number of paramedical personnel per physician has increased from one to four and one half since 1900. Of course, advancing technology may have influenced this. Despite AMA opposition, as chronicled by Rayack (1967), the number of medical personnel in direct competition with physicians has increased greatly since the advent of tight licensing and strict educational standards. Chiropractors for example, have increased by 147 percent from 1940 to 1960, while physicians have increased by only 47 percent (Rayack, 1967, p. 127). In the attempt to substitute less expensive inputs for physicians, hospitals have been led to make more use of residents, the respective numbers of which rose 611 percent from 1940 to 1960 (Rayack, 1967, pp. 123-27).

Similarly, one of the most important results of the entry restrictions of the licensed allied health occupations (which are on average the more skilled health occupations) has been a substitution of lower-skilled manpower for the skilled workers. Based on a careful analysis of Census data, Weiss (1966) calculated that the proportion of health jobs with high skill and income content declined from 34 percent in 1970 to 25 in 1960, while those with low skill and income content rose from 21 to 34 percent. Further, "wage levels for the low-paid hospital jobs have increased more slowly than the wage levels of the higher paid (and usually licensed) technical and professional employees" (Feldstein, 1970, p. 67).

If the numbers of skilled personnel are restricted by licensure, other workers may, as a result, be less productive. Most important, inputs may not be used in correct proportions, thus rendering the medical sector less productive.

Discrimination

Organized medicine's tightening of entry restrictions for physicians had major effects on medical schools. Instead of actively competing for students, medical schools started turning away students in great numbers. Many observers have argued that this state of affairs gave medical schools the ability, for the first time, to discriminate on a large scale against blacks, women, Jews, and other groups in their admissions policy.

As a result of the 1910 Flexner Report and licensing, the number of black medical schools dropped from seven to two, and the number of black students per school also dropped. This had the effect of halting a dramatic increase in the number and percentage of black physicians and ultimately causing a decline. See Tables 6-1 and 6-2.

The peak for the proportion of physicians who were women occurred in 1910. Not only the proportion but the absolute number of women who were physicians was higher in 1910 than 1940 (Shryock, 1950, pp. 371-77).

The question of discrimination against Jews is more complicated. There could have been simply a dislike of Jews, but Kessel argues that Jews are more likely to compete with other doctors because they are culturally different and more difficult to integrate into the "social and economic club" of professional medicine, and because of Jewish attitudes of suspicion of cartels and guilds which make them behave as ". . . robust competitors with little respect for rules, either government or private, that regulate economic activity." During the depression, when admissions to medical schools in general were cut back, Jewish admissions declined by 30 percent, while total admissions declined by only 13 percent (Goldberg, 1939). Further, according to Kessel, virtually all the Americans who study medicine abroad are Jews (1958, pp. 46, 47).

Some evidence of possible discrimination against Jewish medical school applicants is provided in Table 6-3, which shows the percentage of pre-

Table 6-1
Medical Schools, Students, and Graduates: 1905-1960

Year	Schools	Students	Graduates
1905	160	26,147	4,606
1910	131	21,526	4,440–Flexner Report is
1915	104	14,891	3,536 published.
1920	88	14,088	3,047
1925	80	18,200	3,974
1930	76	21,597	4,565–Implementation of
1935	77	22,095	5,101 Flexner Report is
1940	77	21,271	5,097 complete; last unapproved medical
1945	77	24,028	5,136 school is closed.
1950	79	25,103	5,553
1955	81	28,583	6,977
1960	85	30,084	7,081
1965	88	32,428	7,049
1970	101	37,669	8,367

Sources: Rayack (1967, pp. 68-69); *Medical Education in the U.S. 1969-1970*, American Medical Association, 1970; *Health, Education and Welfare Trends, 1966-1967*, U.S. Department of Health, Education, and Welfare, 1967.

Table 6-2
Black Physicians and Physicians of All Races: 1890-1969

Year	Black Physicians	All Physicians	Blacks as a Percent of All Physicians
1890	909	104,805	0.9%
1900	1,734	119,749	1.5
1910	3,409	135,000	2.5—Flexner Report is published
1920	3,855	144,977	2.7 (seven black schools are operating).
1930	3,770	153,803	2.5—Two black medical schools remain.
1940	3,810	165,985	2.2
1950	4,026	191,947	2.1
1960	4,551	260,484[a]	1.8
1969	4,805	338,379	1.4

[a]Osteopaths are included for the first time.

Sources: *Historical Statistics of the United States: Colonial Times to 1957*, Bureau of the Census, 1960, p. 34; *U.S. Census of Population, 1960, Occupational Characteristics*, Bureau of Census, PC(2)-7A, 1961, p. 23; *Statistical Abstract of the United States*, Bureau of Census, 1971, p. 66; Morais (1969, pp. 85, 86, 99, 100, 148, 200).

dominantly Jewish City College of New York applicants who were accepted by medical schools between 1925 and 1943 the percentage of Jews in medical school, no matter how many qualified Jewish applicants were available, was fixed. The mechanism was explained by Dr. Ladd Dean, of the Cornell Medical School, in a letter in 1940 (Bloomgarden, 1953, p. 32):

Cornell Medical College admits a class of eighty each fall . . . from about twelve hundred applicants of whom seven hundred or more are Jews. We limit the (proportion) of Jews admitted to each class to from 10-15 percent.

Thus, a Jew had one chance in seventy of being accepted, while a nonJew had one chance in seven. But, restricting the entry of qualified applicants could be expected to lower the average productivity of the profession.[2]

Table 6-3

Number of (Predominantly Jewish) City College of New York Graduates
Admitted to Medical School: 1929-1943

Year	Number of Applicants	Percentage Admitted
1925	190	58%
1927	205	53
1929	238	29
1932	279	24 – Admissions to medical
1936	189	16 school for all groups
1939	122	15 reduced 13%.
1942	139	16
1943	139	15

Source: Kingdon (1945, p. 394). Reprinted by permission of American Mercury, Box 1306, Torrance, California 90505.

Impact on Medical Education

Many have argued that a major effect of the Flexner Report and subsequent licensing was to set the education of health care workers in a rigid mold; Kessel, in a 1970 article, explains that, until very recently, there has been little experimentation with curricula, teaching methods, and the use of scientists from outside medical schools. Medical education became rigid because of the detailed way in which the AMA, following Flexner, specified the courses and programs required for medical school accreditation, since physicians must have graduated from such an accredited medical school to have been licensed.

The situation is quite similar for allied health manpower. Further, as the HEW report on licensure states (1971, pp. 21-25):

The Council on Medical Education of the American Medical Association is the focal point for the establishment and maintenance of standards of quality and recognition of educational programs meeting these standards (for allied health personnel) . . . (it) now provides accrediting for the following 15 categories of educational programs:

1. Certified Laboratory Assistant
2. Cytotechnologist
3. Histologic Technician
4. Inhalation Therapy Technician
5. Medical Assistant
6. Medical Record Librarian
7. Medical Record Technician
8. Medical Technologist
9. Nuclear Medicine Technician
10. Nuclear Technologist

11. Occupational Therapist
12. Orthopedic Assistant
13. Physical Therapist
14. Radiation Therapy Technologist
15. Radiologic Technologist

It is widely believed that this method of setting education standards retards innovation in medical education. For example, Anthony Robbins writes (1970, p. 60):

... the system discourages new thinking about what a given allied health professional can or cannot do. At a time when medical schools are critically re-examining and changing their curricula, the other health professionals are carefully ossifying their training programs.

Making educational programs more rigid—by tying them to licensure standards—may make them less efficient: fewer professionals are trained, causing substitution away from the professionals as discussed above. Further, inflexible educational patterns may result in the professionals receiving inferior training, further inhibiting productivity.

Prevention of Competition within the Profession

It is often argued that there is a strong tendency for the occupational group itself to gain control of the licensure mechanism.[3] A majority of health occupation licensing authorities are composed *entirely* of members of the occupation (Pennell and Stewart, 1967, p. 10). Further, the revocation of a license can be used as a sanction to enable a profession to discourage behavior which benefits an individual member, but which harms the profession as a whole. There are gains which the profession can obtain by restricting competition among those who are allowed to enter it. Kessel (1958), Rayack (1967) and M. Friedman (1962, Ch. IX) argue that each professional can earn more if his customers are as isolated as possible from competing workers, both because he can charge higher fees or be paid a higher salary, and because he can price-discriminate if he is an independent practitioner.[4]

The methods of limiting internal competition discussed by Kessel, Rayack, and M. Friedman include prohibitions of advertising and opposition to new forms of prepaid group practice. These observers report that licensure and hospital privileges were the sanctions most often used.

Competition and Mobility among Occupations and Specialties

Greenfield (1969, p. 101) believes that the defense of jurisdictional areas among health occupations leads to

. . . jurisdictional disputes between contiguous groups such as the LPN (Licensed Practical Nurse) and RN (Registered Nurse), the medical technicians and technologists, and even the RN and the MD. These inter-occupational disputes . . . not only are the source of friction among workers, but are also the cause of malutilization of hospital manpower.[5]

The main weapon in each jurisdictional joust seems to be occupational licensure. In the allied health occupations, this jurisdictional restrictionism is widely thought to have seriously restricted upward and lateral mobility. The DHEW licensure report notes that licensure processes "often operate in such a way as to 'lock-in' individuals to certain positions with little potential for the assumption of increased responsibility or mobility" (1971, p. 99). For example, there are three skill levels of nurses (nurses aid, Licensed Practical Nurse, and Registered Nurse). If one desired to rise from one level to another, one would be required to take the entire training program for each level, with no prior training or experience counting toward the requirements of each grade.

The ruling bodies of the AMA and the American Hospital Association have criticized licensing for paramedical personnel and called for wider rights of physicians to delegate tasks to paramedical personnel (AMA, 1970; AHA, 1971).[6] The AMA states:

. . . there is need to avoid the problems of overspecialization and fractionalization of services entailed by occupational licensure systems and the resultant controls on entry into occupations and scope of permissible functions . . . *There seems to be a growing body of opinion that occupational licensure has outlived its usefulness as a method assuring quality health services.*
   Proliferation in mandatory occupational licensure laws tends to foster a "craft union" approach to health care and may lead to unwarranted increase in cost of services . . .
   Current occupational licensure laws tend to inhibit innovation in the education and use of allied health manpower and restrict the avenues available for entry into or upward mobility in a health career . . . (emphasis in original).

This view is echoed, in a slightly milder form, by the American Hospital Association (1971) and by many observers (Forgotson and Cook, 1967; Hershey, 1969).

However, far-reaching reforms may meet difficult legal problems. According to the legal analysis of Forgotson and Cook (1967, p. 735), licensure for semiindependent health workers is virtually required by the existence of licensing for physicians. When physician licensure was made mandatory, it became necessary to define the practice of medicine. The definitions were very broad and included all personal health services. Thus, new categories of health occupations which function under indirect physician supervision (or no supervision at all) must be licensed by carrying out limited exceptions to broad physician licenses.

There are also serious jurisdictional disputes within the medical profession itself—in the form of disputes among specialists and between specialists and general practitioners:

... general practitioners battle specialists and various types of specialists battle one another as each group is engaged in an imperialistic struggle to protect or expand its domain over segments of the human anatomy (Rayack, 1967, p. 202).

Since licensing laws for physicians makes no mention of specialties, any physician can treat any malady using his own facilities. The disputes, then, have centered over the issue of hospital privileges, a kind of restriction which is quite common. A 1962 survey showed that most hospitals limit privileges for general practitioners (Rayack, 1967, pp. 221-222). Dr. Charles E. Letourneau, President of the College of Legal Medicine, explained the occasional loss of hospital privileges by general practitioners (Rayack, 1967, p. 224):

Yes, typically this happens when a horde of surgical specialists moves into an area only to discover there's not enough surgery around. I've seen it affect four or five hospitals in the same community. Board-certified men tried to freeze out the competition completely, although local G.P.'s have been there for thirty years doing good work.

Since specialty board membership often implies greater access to important hospital facilities, it is a sort of quasilicense, enabling the member to practice medicine on a certain part of the anatomy. It is in the interest of the existing specialties if membership is restricted. Stevens and Vermuelen have examined the methods which the various specialty boards have adopted to restrict entry. Several specialty boards require applicants to be U.S. citizens. The specialty boards for dermatology, internal medicine and orthopedic surgery certify foreign medical graduates only if they are leaving the country. They must *surrender their certification* if they return to the U.S. The board of neurological surgery does not certify foreigners: it only "authenticates" them if they pass all the tests and meet all the requirements for certification. A number of boards require letters of recommendation for certified specialists in the applicant's home community. The boards of anesthesiology and ophthamology reserve the right to limit the number of applicants who may take the examination at any one time (Stevens and Vermuelen, 1971, p. III-18).

Geographical Mobility Restrictions

The use of licensure to restrict the immigration of qualified professionals is a very common phenomenon which seems to be in the interest of the professions and contrary to that of consumers. Barriers of this type seem to be least common for U.S.-trained physicians and most important for foreign-trained professionals, especially paramedical personnel. Forty-eight states and the District of Columbia license physicians who were licensed in other states by either endorsement[7] or reciprocity with the original licensing state. The exceptions are states which are experiencing rapid population growth—Florida and Hawaii. In these states, an immigrant must take an examination to be licensed.

As an example of allied health personnel, dental hygienists have much less reciprocity. Only 12 states maintain such agreements for them (Council on Dental Education, 1970, p. 2).

The U.S. is an attractive place to train foreigners because of high salary levels. There are higher and more universal barriers against foreigners in each American state than the barriers against members of the occupation from another state. Of course, the strongest barrier against foreign-trained health workers is simply not to license them at all. Five states do not license foreign physicians (Derbyshire, 1969, pp. 143, 145); several states exclude physical therapists, veterinarians and other health occupations, and *no state* licenses dental hygienists who were educated outside the U.S. (Pennell and Stewart, 1967, pp. 17, 18). Many state licensing agencies require additional training in the U.S. *after* foreign training. Seventeen states require more clinical (internship and residency) experience for foreign medical graduates than for U.S. graduates. Several states require additional tests of foreign-trained health workers educated in countries other than the U.S. or Canada. Three states require a basic science exam and seven require oral exams only for foreign-trained physicians. Five states require foreign medical graduates to be residents of the state for periods ranging from 60 days to five years. Twenty-one states require actual citizenship, while twenty are satisfied with legal declaration of intent to file for citizenship (Pennell and Stewart, 1967, p. 117).

After a foreign-trained person has overcome extraordinary obstacles to become licensed in one state, his mobility is more limited than that of his American-educated counterpart. Most American states license physicians from another state on a reciprocal basis. However, in the case of foreign medical graduates, only thirteen states have this policy. In the rest, the migrant must take another test (Derbyshire, 1969, p. 143).

One of the major obstacles to licensure of physicians educated overseas is the requirement that they pass the examination of the Educational Council for Foreign Medical Graduates (ECFMG) before they are admitted to internship in the United States. Since internship is a prerequisite for licensure, this examination forms an important barrier to entry. The ECFMG was set up in 1956 to evaluate the training of foreign medical graduates after the AMA's attempt to evaluate foreign medical schools, as they do for U.S. schools, was given up as too complex.

The ECFMG and its exam could not prohibit hospitals and other institutions from hiring foreign graduates as interns and residents. The demand was great and the supply small. Teeth were put into the ECFMG exam by a 1960 AMA policy which stated that no hospital could retain its approved internship and residency programs if it used interns who were not approved by the ECFMG. Since internship in an approved program is necessary to obtain a license, this new rule effectively used the licensing power to exclude many foreign graduates. Implementation of the exam program was complete by 1966. Since then, passing rates for foreign graduates have averaged around 40 percent at one sitting (Stevens and Vermeulen, 1971, p. III-6).

Hospital administrators were, as might be expected, unhappy about the exclusion of those who failed the exam. A New York hospital administrator said:

The ECFMG should simply publish the results and let the hospital decide whether it wants a man who got a score of, say, 50. In my opinion it's better to have a poorly-trained intern than no intern at all.[8]

Stevens and Vermeulen (1971) reported on the way organized medicine has attempted to reduce permanent and temporary immigration of foreign-trained medical personnel. A report of a House of Representatives Subcommittee of the Committee on the Judiciary recommended the formalization of existing preferential treatment of medical graduates and the increasing freedom for medical graduates of foreign countries to immigrate (temporarily and permanently) into the U.S. (Report of Subcommittee No. 1, 1970).

The AMA strongly opposed admitting physicians into the U.S. to fill hospital demand for personnel. The AMA also supported the provision of the law requiring, for certain classes of medical immigrants, a two-year stay abroad before returning to the U.S., encouraged foreign physicians to return to their homeland and opposed the existing use of waivers to allow them to stay longer in the U.S. (Stevens and Vermeulen, 1971).

In 1965, Congress amended the Immigration Act to make physician immigration easier by allowing preference for professionals and those with skills in "shortage" occupations. Physicians fit into both categories, as the amended act is being administered. The law was liberalized still more in 1970, as American legislators believed that the physician "shortage" could be alleviated by the admission of more foreign physicians.

However, not all movement has been in the direction of free migration. Pressure on the Labor Department by the ECFMG, the AMA, and the American Association of Medical Colleges has resulted in new rules requiring that the potential physician immigrant prove before admission to the U.S. that (Stevens and Vermeulen, 1971, p. III-10):

1. He has met licensure requirements or requirements to take the licensing examination in the state within which he intends to practice, or

2. He has met the requirements for and has been offered an AMA approved internship or residency, or
3. He has passed the ECFMG examination, or
4. His appointment does not involve direct physician care.

There is a possibility that discrimination against foreign medical graduates may be struck down by the courts. Eight hundred American students studying at Guadalajara (Mexico) University filed suit against the ECFMG and the professional organizations for violation of constitutional rights, antitrust infractions, and conspiracy (Stevens and Vermeulen, 1971, Ch. III).

In spite of these obstacles, in many states foreign medical graduates are apparently, on average, less well prepared than U.S. graduates. This anomaly has arisen because the main entry restriction, control of medical education, cannot be easily applied to foreign graduates.

In a recent year, the failure rate on state licensure examinations was about four percent for U.S.-trained physicians versus 40 percent for those educated abroad (Derbyshire, 1969, p. 142). Of course, some of this difference may be due to language problems and/or different educational emphasis, unrelated to professional competence. But these geographical restrictions reduce average productivity by keeping health professionals in states where they are already relatively oversupplied.

Some Policy Issues

As Friedman argues (1962, Ch. IX), a system of certification might provide all the informational advantages of licensure without the restrictive opportunities for the professions (assuming minimal consumer learning ability). However, the idea of replacing the current licensure system with one of certification in licensed health professions might be very threatening and politically unrealistic. Less sweeping policy proposals which promise reductions in the restrictive power of licensure, and therefore promise gains in productivity, may be more feasible.

Professor Hershey has proposed "An Alternative to Mandatory Licensure of Health Professionals" (1969, p. 71). His alternative is "institutional licensure"— licensing of the health care institutions, making them responsible for quality. In effect, this simply ends licensure of allied health personnel, transforming existing licensure programs into certification programs. Hershey applies this plan to private physician practice by suggesting that "the individual physician's office be recognized as a small health care institution" (p. 74). Hershey's plan would reverse the restrictions said to be caused by licensure, but would maintain the information-providing features of certification. Of course, institutional licensure may itself become restrictive, but that seems less serious because each institution could expand output.

Another policy idea which aims at reform of licensure rather than its replacement has been set forth by Kessel (1970, p. 19). He proposes to transform state licensure examinations into more meaningful ones by opening them up to all comers, regardless of how they acquired their skills. Thus, licensure would be defined by *output* in terms of skills and knowledge, rather than by *inputs* in terms of educational and professional experience. Medical education would then be entirely free to experiment and discover the most productive methods of imparting the necessary skills rather than remaining tied to traditional methods spelled out by licensing agencies. The potential for increased productivity here is apparent. Recently, with DHEW prodding and support, there have been experiments with such proficiency testing as a basis for licensure and Medicare qualifications. Several professions have been involved, the largest of which is physical therapy (*Report on Licensure* . . . , 1971, pp. 111-13).

A second part of Kessel's plan is to require periodical relicensure based on the same or a very similar test. This feature would prevent examinations from becoming too restrictive, since existing practitioners could be excluded as well as newcomers; also, by weeding out some of the worst physicians who are already practicing, it would probably increase the average quality of American physicians, and truly raise productivity. This plan makes entry into the medical profession easier because it is totally proficiency based. At the same time, it eliminates those physicians who are very bad and would not be affected by current licensure. Thus, it might provide both better quality protection and freer entry. Further, Kessel argues that this relicensure program would reduce much of the power of organized medicine over existing members of the profession. Most of this power is based on control of approved internship programs, and thus hospitals and hospital privileges. If there were no longer any formalized educational requirements, organized medicine could no longer threaten to withhold interns from (and thus control) hospitals. Thus, Kessel would expect to see more freedom for practitioners to compete, with lower prices for better medical care.

Of course, these proposals could also be applied to nonphysician manpower, with similar expectations.

Suggested Research

Thus far, much of the research on occupational licensure in the health field has been either application of economic theory or anecdotal historical studies. While these have been both interesting and illuminating, the need for empirically based research on the magnitudes of the various effects which have been observed is increasingly apparent.

There are three main types of quantitative studies which would be very useful: time series analysis, cross sectional analysis, and empirically based simulations.

Time Series

Natural and important research might examine the various professions as they have progressed over time. Since the typical profession has moved from more or less complete free entry to various stages of licensure within the past eighty years (and generally a much shorter period of time), one could analyze the relationship between the time path of licensure strictness and a number of economic variables such as the number of practitioners, average schooling, average incomes and the behavior of substitute inputs such as closely related professions. This would allow estimates of the increase in costs of care (if any) attributable to licensure. Further, for professions which are very uniform across states in licensure requirements (e.g., physicians), this time series approach is the only method to *directly* estimate some of the impacts of licensure.

Cross Section

For some professions, there is a great deal of variation across states in the degree of licensure strictness and in the length of time which any degree of strictness has been maintained. This allows the estimation of the effects of licensure on similar economic variables to those discussed above for professions across states at a point in time.

Where it is possible, this approach is likely to be much more effective than the time series methods because of the difficulty in separating the independent effort of licensure (or any other single economic variable), as many variables move together over time. Aside from this multicolinearity problem which is intrinsic in the data, there are statistical problems which often arise in estimation with time series data, such as serial correlation of errors. Also, technological conditions are (especially in medicine) changing very rapidly, so that the comparability of American medicine over time is somewhat difficult to interpret. Cross-sectional estimation allows one to hold technology relatively constant.

As a variant of cross sectional analysis, one could compare *different* professions which were adjudged to be more or less similar but which vary in licensure. Clearly this is quite difficult to interpret (as are cross-industry studies in the industrial organization literature), but for professions which are nationally uniform but which have a short history, this is the only method of direct estimation of effects.

Simulation

The advantage of simulation methods is that they allow one to make use of noneconometric information, of both an industrial engineering sort and from other industries, to examine the effects of changes in licensure regulations on medical markets. This permits the estimation of relationships for which there is too little direct data to directly estimate relationships.

As an example, one might combine industrial engineering data about the productivity of, say, unrestricted physician's assistants with data on the market wages in other industries of people with similar degrees of (different) skill, to simulate the impact of nonlicensed, unrestricted physicians' assistants. Combining that information with empirical estimates of supply and demand elasticities, one could predict the impact of free entry into such a profession in terms of the cost of care, the distribution of care, the incomes of other health professionals, and so on.

In general, the more-or-less radical kinds of policy changes, such as discussed above, can only be investigated by some kind of simulation model. An important consideration which has been ignored in some recent simulation efforts is to make as much use as possible of empirically estimated parameters rather than assumptions of parameter values.

Notes

1. For a discussion of this point for licensure in general, see Gellhorn (1956) and Stigler (1971).

2. For more complete references to the extensive literature on anti-Semitic discrimination in medical schools, see Kessel (1958, 1970).

3. According to Gellhorn (1956, p. 140):

Seventy-five percent of the occupational licensing boards . . . in this country are composed exclusively of licensed practitioners in the respective occupations. These men and women . . . may have a direct economic interest in many of the decisions they make . . . More importantly, they are, as a rule, directly representative of organized groups within the occupation. Ordinarily, they are nominated by these groups as a step toward . . . appointment that is frequently a mere formality. Often the formality is dispensed with entirely, appointment being made directly by the occupational association—as happens with the embalmers in North Carolina, the psychologists in Virginia, the physicians in Maryland, and the attorneys in Washington.

4. Although price discrimination *per se* is not inefficient, it is a sign that providers individually are significantly isolated from competition, and professional efforts to preserve price discrimination may reduce competition and promote efficiency.

5. Greenfield (1969, p. 155) cites the pathologists who so strenuously attempted to prevent chemists and biochemists from operating clinical laboratories that the Justice Department sued for restraint of trade.

6. See also Ruth Roemer (1971).

7. Endorsement means granting a license on the assumption that the standards in the original licensing state are equivalent to the receiving state.

8. Quoted by Stevens and Vermeulen (1971, p. III-7).

Bibliography

American Hospital Association, "Statement on Licensure of Health Care Personnel," *Hospitals, Journal of the American Hospital Association*, Vol. 45 (March 16, 1971).

American Medical Association, "Licensure of Health Occupations," Adopted by House of Delegates (December 1970).

Becker, Gary S., *Human Capital*, New York: National Bureau of Economic Research, 1964.

Beckman, Jules, *Advertising and Competition*. New York: New York University Press, 1967.

Benham, Lee, "The Effect of Advertising on the Price of Eyeglasses," *Journal of Law and Economics*, Vol. 15, No. 2 (October 1972), pp. 337-52.

Bevan, A.D., "Cooperation in Medical Education and Medical Service," *Journal of the American Medical Society*, Vol. 90 (1928).

Bloomgarden, Lawrence, "Medical School Quotas and National Health," *Commentary*, Vol. 15, No. 1 (January 1953), pp. 29-37.

Council on Dental Education, American Dental Association, *Requirements and Registration Data: Dental Hygiene* (1970).

Derbyshire, Robert C., M.D., *Medical Licensure and Discipline in the United States*. Baltimore: The Johns Hopkins Press, 1969.

Educational Council for Foreign Medical Graduates, *Annual Report* (1969).

Feldstein, Martin S., "The Rising Cost of Hospital Care," unpublished paper, Harvard University (July 30, 1970).

Forgotson, Edward H., and John L. Cook, "Innovations and Experiments in Uses of Health Manpower—The Effect of Licensure Laws," *Law and Contemporary Problems*, Vol. 32 (Autumn 1967), pp. 731-50.

Friedman, Lawrence M., "Freedom of Contracts and Occupational Licensing, 1890-1910, A Legal and Social Study," *California Law Review*, Vol. 53, No. 2 (May 1965).

Friedman, Milton, *Capitalism and Freedom*. Chicago: University of Chicago Press, 1962.

Friedman, Milton, and Simon Kuznets. *Income from Independent Professional Practice*. New York: National Bureau of Economic Research, 1945.

Gellhorn, Walter, *Individual Freedom and Governmental Restraints*. Baton Rouge: Louisiana State University Press, 1956.

Goldberg, Jacob A., "Jews in the Medical Profession—A National Survey," *Jewish Social Studies*, Vol. 1, No. 3 (July 1939), pp. 327-66.

Greenfield, Harry I., *Allied Health Manpower: Trends and Prospects*, New York: Columbia University Press, 1969, pp. 155-157.

Hearings Before Subcommittee No. 1 of the Committee on the Judiciary House of Representatives, 91st Congress, 2nd Session, on H.R. 9112, H.R. 15092,

H.R. 17370: To Amend the Immigration and Nationality Act, and for Other Purposes (July 16, 22, 29, August 5, 6, 1970).

Hershey, Nathan, "An Alternative to Mandatory Licensure of Health Professionals," *Hospital Progress*, Vol. 50 (March 1969), pp. 71-74.

Kessel, Reuben A., "The AMA and the Supply of Physicians," *Law and Contemporary Problems*, Health Care Pt. 1, Vol. 35, No. 2, (Spring 1970), pp. 267-83.

_____, "Price Discrimination in Medicine," *Journal of Law and Economics*, Vol. 1 (October 1958), pp. 20-54.

Kingdon, Frank, "Discrimination in Medical Colleges," *American Mercury*, Vol. 61, No. 262 (October 1945), pp. 391-99.

Kolko, Gabriel, *The Triumph of Conservatism*. Chicago: Quadrangle Books, 1967.

Konold, Donald E., *A History of American Medical Ethics, 1846-1912*. State Historical Society of Wisconsin for the Department of History, University of Wisconsin, Madison, 1962.

"Medical Licensure Statistics—1969," *Journal of the American Medical Association*, Vol. 212, No. 11 (June 15, 1970), p. 1925.

Moore, T. Gale, "The Purpose of Licensing," *Journal of Law and Economics*, Vol. 4 (October 1961), pp. 93-117.

Morais, Herbert M., *The History of the Negro in Medicine*. New York: Publishers Co., 1969.

National Advisory Commission on Health Manpower, *Report of the National Advisory Commission on Health Manpower*. Washington, D.C.: U.S. Government Printing Office, 1967.

Owens, Arthur, "Inflation Closes in on Physicians' Earnings," *Medical Economics* (December 21, 1970), pp. 63-71.

Peltzman, Sam, "Entry in Commercial Banking," *Journal of Law and Economics*, Vol. 8 (October 1965), pp. 11-50.

Pennell, Maryland Y., and Paula A. Stewart, *State Licensing of Health Occupations*. Washington, D.C.: U.S. Government Printing Office, Public Health Service Publication No. 1758, 1967.

Rayack, Elton, *Professional Power and American Medicine: The Economics of the American Medical Association*. New York: World, 1967.

Report on Licensure and Related Health Personnel Credentialing. Office of the Assistant Secretary for Health and Scientific Affairs, Department of Health, Education, and Welfare, Washington, D.C. (June 1971).

Robbins, Anthony, "Allied Health Manpower," *Inquiry*, Vol. 7, No. 1 (March 1970), p. 55-61.

Roemer, Ruth, "Licensing and Regulation of Medical and Medical-related Practitioners in Health Service Teams," *Medical Care*, Vol. 9, No. 1 (January/February 1971), pp. 42-54.

Rottenberg, Simon, "Economics of Occupational Licensing," in *Aspects of Labor Economics*, NBER. Princeton: Princeton University Press, 1962.

Shryock, Richard Harrison, *Medical Licensing in America, 1950-1965*. Baltimore: The Johns Hopkins Press, 1967.

———, "Women in American Medicine," *Journal of the American Women's Medical Association*, Vol. 5 (1950), pp. 371-77.

Sloan, Frank A., "Lifetime Earnings and Physician's Choice of Specialty," *Industrial and Labor Relations*, Vol. 24, No. 1 (October 1970), pp. 47-56.

Stevens, Rosemary, and Jean Vermeulen, "Foreign-Trained Physicians and American Medicine," unpublished paper, Yale University, June 1971.

Stigler, George J., "The Economics of Information," *Journal of Political Economy*, Vol. 69, No. 3 (June 1961), pp. 213-225.

———, "The Theory of Regulation," *Bell Journal of Economics and Management Science*, Vol. 2, No. 1 (Spring 1971), pp. 3-21.

Todd, C., and M.E. McNamara, *Survey of Medical Groups in the United States, 1969*. Chicago: American Medical Association, 1971.

Weiss, Jeffrey H., *The Changing Structure of Health Manpower*, unpublished Ph.D. dissertation, Harvard University, 1966.

West, Kelly M., M.D., "Some Opinions and Myths Concerning Foreign Medical Graduates," *Federation Bulletin*, Vol. 56, No. 12, pp. 338-52.

Yett, Donald E., "Causes and Consequences of Salary Differentials in Nursing," *Inquiry*, Vol. 7, No. 1 (March 1970), pp. 78-99.

Part II
A General Overview

Research on Health Manpower Productivity: A General Overview

Jack Hadley*

Introduction

Economics and economists have traditionally devoted their energies to analyzing the general problem of how to allocate society's scarce resources so as to satisfy, to as great an extent as possible, the various wants of the population. The questions representing this task are familiar: What goods and services should be produced? How should scarce resources be combined to produce these goods and services? And, who is to receive the outputs of the production process? Although these questions are usually framed at the economy-wide or national level, they are equally appropriate (with some modifications) at both larger and smaller units of analysis.[1] Thus, they are also relevant for the health services sector.

The first asks whether we are producing the proper mix of health services. Do we have the "right" configuration of hospital services and ambulatory services, of mental health care and convalescent care, of surgical procedures and physical therapy programs, etc.?[2] Next, given the mix of outputs we want to produce, are we producing them efficiently? Could we get greater output of health services for the same amount of inputs, or, conversely, could we produce the same output using fewer inputs? Finally, how and to whom should health services be distributed? The first two questions may be thought of as primarily efficiency-oriented, while the last is a matter of equity.

As the concept of productivity implies, its main focal point is in the production process, i.e., the way in which inputs are combined to produce the various outputs of the health sector. It will be shown below that changes in the mix of outputs produced or in the distribution of health services to recipients can also have an effect on manpower productivity. However, in dealing explicitly with productivity, we shall look primarily at the relationship between inputs and outputs in producing health services, without asking if this is necessarily the best mix of services, or if they are being optimally distributed.

Definitions

While there are many notions about what productivity is, the concept has a

*Economist, Bureau of Health Services Research and Evaluation.

143

precise definition within economics, and to state this definition, it would be useful to adopt a small amount of formalism. Think of health services as the end result of combining various quantities of health manpower, capital, and other medical inputs in accordance with some set of technological relations. A convenient representation of these relationships is provided by the notion of the "production function," which can be simply expressed in mathematical notation as

$$Q = f(L_1, \ldots, L_n; K; M; T).\tag{7.1}$$

In this expression, Q is the quantity of health services produced; the L_i represent the various health manpower inputs, e.g., L_1 may be the input of physician person-hours, L_2 of nurse person-hours, L_3 of ancillary person-hours, etc.; K is a vector of the different types of capital inputs such as buildings, office equipment, lab equipment, beds, etc.; M is also a vector, representing other medical inputs such as disposables, laundry and food services, bandages, drugs, etc., which are used in producing health services; and, finally, T denotes the technology being employed.

This representation is extremely general, in that it does not indicate either the exact way in which the inputs are combined (i.e., the functional form is not specified), the nature of the output being produced, or the practice or organizational setting in which production takes place. One might formulate a separate production function for every type of medical procedure or service, or one could combine outputs and inputs into an *aggregate* production function. In either case the definition of productivity remains the same. Very simply, productivity is defined as "output per unit of input." The key questions here, then, are: (1) what are the proper theoretical concepts of health services inputs and outputs, and (2) how may they be measured?

With regard to inputs, one common approach is to focus on the productivity of the physician. In this case, (continuing with the above notation) if L_1 represents the quantity of physician-hours (of a specified kind) involved in the production process, productivity is defined as the ratio:

$$Q/L_1 = \frac{f(L_1, \ldots, L_n; K; M; T)}{L_1}.\tag{7.2}$$

This is usually justified on the grounds that the physician is the central and most important type of health manpower, the most scarce, and also the most expensive. In the same way one could define the productivity of other manpower inputs such as nurses, ancillaries, technicians, etc., as:

$$Q/L_i = \frac{f(L_1, \ldots, L_n; K; M; T)}{L_i}, \qquad i = 2, \ldots, n.\tag{7.3}$$

It should be clear, of course, that we could similarly define the productivity of capital or of any of the other production function inputs as well.

Alternatively, one might be concerned with the productivity of total health manpower. Ideally, production inputs are measured in physical units. In order to make this productivity measure meaningful, one must first devise a method of combining the heterogeneous inputs into a single index. The approach most frequently used is to weigh each type of input by its price (wage or salary). For example, we might create the index P, defined as:

$$P = W_1 L_1 + W_2 L_2 + \ldots + W_n L_n, \tag{7.4}$$

Where W_i = price of the ith input. Therefore, manpower productivity would now be defined as:

$$Q/P = \frac{f(L_1, \ldots, L_n; K; M; T)}{P}. \tag{7.5}$$

There are, however, some difficulties with this approach. First, the price of a physician is very difficult to define conceptually, and almost impossible to measure empirically. Secondly, this particular way of defining productivity is less useful for policy purposes because it does not allow us to identify which specific types of health manpower have increased their productivity.

Regardless of which input is chosen, measurement is relatively straightforward. Fairly good head-counts of health manpower are available, and, with the exception of physicians, relatively good information on salaries is also available.[3] This is not the case, however, for hospitals and hospital production functions, since no one has yet been able to determine or measure physicians' contributions to hospital output.

The definition and measurement of output, however, is far more ambiguous. It has often been argued that the proper theoretical concept of output of the health services industry should be health itself, or at least the change in health due to the use of medical care services. This implies looking at such variables as mortality rates, morbidity rates, number of disability days, or some index of overall health status. While intuitively appealing, this approach is rejected here for several reasons. First, designating health as the output of the production function specified in Equation (7.1) would require adding to the right-hand side of the equation a number of inputs which have little or nothing to do with health services delivery. Levels of food consumption, housing, hygiene, nutrition, highway and automobile safety, alcoholism and drug addiction, etc., immediately come to mind as examples of nonmedical services which can have a profound effect on health. Further, both the measurement of some of these variables and the specification of the nature of the technical relationships between them and health would be extremely difficult. On the other hand, if one leaves these factors out of the production function, the effect of medical inputs on health is overstated, and this might tend to lead to a misallocation of policy emphasis, away from these "environmental" factors towards the more explicit and more easily measurable medical inputs.[4]

One might represent the idealized health production function by the scheme below. Health is seen to be a function of a number of factors, including medical treatments, represented by the boxes, A, B, C, and D.

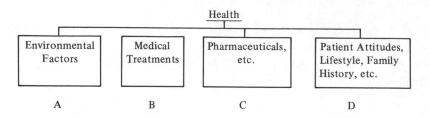

We could presumably disaggregate each of the boxes into its constituent parts, designate which factors are exogenous (beyond the individual's control), endogenous, or represent technical or institutional constraints and, finally, we could specify the set of interrelationships of these variables with health and with each other. Assuming everything were measurable, the contribution of each variable could then be estimated.

Clearly this is an impossible task at this time. Therefore, as a proximate solution to this dilemma, we usually concentrate on medical treatments as the output of the health services industry. In breaking this box down, we could think in terms of the types of care patients receive (e.g., inpatient or ambulatory, long-term or short-term) or, alternatively, we could focus on the institution delivering care (e.g., the private practice physician, the short-term hospital, the clinic or group practices, etc.). This approach suggests variables such as patient contacts or visits, patient days, admission rates, illness episodes, medical procedures, etc., as candidates for output measures. The key assumption which must be made to justify this approach is that increased quantities of health services outputs improve health. It then follows that increased efficiency in the production of health services (caused by, say, increases in health manpower productivity) enables society to achieve a higher health status level for a given expenditure of scarce resources.

There is still the problem of selecting an output definition from among the set of intermediate variables. Each has somewhat different implications and provides different incentives for behavior. For example, suppose physicians were reimbursed on the basis of patient visits as opposed to, say, illness episodes. And suppose further that the patient visit was also our proxy output measure for studying physician productivity. Clearly, physicians' financial incentives could then lead to an increased "fractionation" of illness episodes,[5] thereby indicating an artificial increase in output for the same input levels—i.e., an increase in measured productivity.

A second problem which arises is that the intermediate output definitions suggested above represent a highly heterogeneous mix of services and activities. One solution to this problem is to study manpower productivity only at very disaggregated levels of analysis, chosen such that the outputs of the production function are by their nature homogeneous. Thus, for example, one might specify lab tests per lab technician, deliveries per obstetrician, or eye refractions per optometrist as the relevant productivity measures in a series of microeconomic analyses. If, however, we are interested in productivity at a more aggregate level, the hospital, group practice, or state health system, for example, then this approach would not be very satisfactory. The alternative is to define an output index analogous to the index of manpower inputs described above. This would imply taking all the services produced by hospital physicians, or all services produced by physicians in private practice, and then weighting them so as to create a single output measure.

The next relevant question, of course, is what weights should be used. The economist's first response would most likely be to employ the prices charged as weights. In effect, this is what is done when output is specified in monetary rather than physical terms. For goods which are exchanged in a competitive (or at least nearly competitive) market, this choice of weights is quite appropriate. Under certain conditions (namely, those associated with a perfectly competitive market), it can be argued that the prices simultaneously represent both the costs of the resources employed in producing the good or service, and also the good's worth to the consumer.

Unfortunately, these assumptions tend not to hold in the medical care sector, for two major reasons. One is the consumer's (patient's) relative ignorance of the nature of the good which he is buying. To a large extent, patient ignorance has led to the now well-known agency relationship between patients and physicians, who in effect have become the relevant demanders of medical services. Given that the physician is the relevant demander, it is very likely the case that his/her choices and valuations of medical care may be very different from those which an *informed* patient might make. The second major difficulty in employing prices is caused by the ubiquitousness of insurance. In general, the presence of insurance will cause distortions in the set of treatments which providers decide to offer, the prices charged for them, and their utilization by patients. While all such responses may be consistent with rational behavior, the observed price weights of an output index would not be likely to possess the normative characteristics of prices generated in a competitive market.

It should be apparent that the issues inherent in defining and measuring output are crucial to any discussion of manpower productivity. However, to discuss these matters at the level of detail they require would exceed the scope of this chapter. Our purpose here is only to highlight them as problems which must be kept in mind in the ensuing discussion. We may conclude, however, that determination of a proper set of output weights should be a major research objective.

One approach which is relevant to this objective is the development of relative value scales. For example, studies by Hughes et al. (1972, 1973) employed the California Relative Value Scale (CRVS) to weight various types of surgical operations in order to create a measure of surgeon output. Essentially, the weights for operations are based upon the average amount of time required for each type of surgical procedure. While this is certainly a step in the right direction, the CRVS weights (and any other weights based on time inputs) still neglect the patient's or consumer's valuations of the services provided. Further, the CRVS specifically warns against making comparisons across medical specialties, implying that their utility is limited to the disaggregated types of studies mentioned above.

Alternatively, we might consider strengthening market mechanisms in the medical care sector. This would require both restructuring insurance schemes so as to minimize distortions, and, secondly, increasing patient knowledge so that more informed decisions would be possible.

Caveats

Thus far nothing has been said of the quality of care or the quality and skill of health manpower inputs. How does quality enter into the notion of a production function? How does quality affect attempts to analyze health manpower productivity? What can be said about maintaining quality levels, or about changing quality? These questions are all of considerable importance.

Many physicians, hospital administrators, other health professionals, and much of the general population feel that attaining and maintaining the highest quality care for all should be one of the objectives of the health sector and public policy. This is understandable, given the fact that the health care system can be described as an "anxiety-driven" system.[6] Most people seek medical care because of pain, possible disability, or emotional discomfort. At the same time, health professionals are imbued with the moral, ethical, legal, and human consequences of their actions. Further, some recent and spectacular breakthroughs in medicine (heart transplants and hemodialysis for example) have greatly increased public expectations of both the efficacy and availability of medical care.

Unfortunately, many do not realize that medical advances have been less than dramatic in many fields, that there is still much about disease etiology, growth, and transmission which is not known, and that many of the "medical miracles" are extremely expensive and not always clearly beneficial. (Consider, for example, the average survival times of post-heart transplant patients and the recent evidence regarding the effectiveness of ICUs in heart attack patients' survival rates.[7]) If one takes the "highest quality of care" to mean the best techniques and highest professional standards currently operative, then the cost implications of extending this level of care to the entire population are enormous. An example of this is the estimated cost of one billion dollars per year of providing hemodialysis to all people with malfunctioning kidneys.[8] It is highly likely, in fact, that an across-the-board application of the best practice potential would entail a resource cost far higher than society would be willing to incur.

The implication, obviously, is that quality objectives will have to be framed in terms of either some minimally acceptable level of quality or an average quality level. Determination of these levels will depend not only on professional standards, but also on the value society assigns to health and the quantity of resources it is willing to allocate to health services. We must also remember that in a world of scarce resources there are tradeoffs between the distribution of medical care, the total quantity of services provided, and medical care quality. Providing some medical care, albeit of possibly lower quality, may be preferable to an alternative of no medical care whatsoever. These too are social-political decisions which lie beyond the scope of this chapter. The relevant point, though, is that suggested policies which might increase manpower productivity at the possible cost of some reduction in quality should not necessarily be rejected out of hand.

In addition to the value judgments associated with decisions regarding the quality of care, there are also the technical problems of how to incorporate quality levels and quality changes into an analysis of health manpower productivity. One possibility is to assume that quality remains constant over the proposed range of productivity increasing policies. For example, if one were interested in analyzing assembly line productivity in the manufacture of Cadillac, Lincoln, and Chrysler automobiles, then the assumption of relatively constant quality, both from model to model and year to year (as long as the time period is not too long) would not seem to violate reality. Such an assumption, however, would clearly not be appropriate for the medical care sector. Output is highly heterogeneous and difficult to identify, and the sector itself is very dynamic, continually evolving and diffusing new levels of technology, knowledge, and quality.

We might next ask what economists have done in other markets characterized by rapid technological and quality change. Traditionally, the assumption has been made that movements in output *prices* capture improvement (or deterioration) in product quality. This implies that rather than looking at physical measures of output in order to analyze productivity, one should instead focus on the market value (price X quantity) of output. This would be appropriate, for example, in a study of television set production. Here the problem is how to account for the higher quality of color TV sets over black and white receivers.

Clearly, a simple count of all sets produced would underestimate true output levels. Looking at the relative prices of the two kinds of receivers, however, indicates that a color TV set is worth approximately two black and white TVs. Our current assumption would imply that although there are several factors which contribute to the difference in prices, quality difference is certainly one of them, and is captured in the higher price of a color TV.[9]

One could take account of differences in input quality in very much the same way, i.e., by looking at relative input prices. Thus, if two machines performed the same function, but one is less likely to break down or make errors, then its price would be higher, presumably reflecting its higher quality. Similarly, variations in manpower skills and quality would be indicated, in part, by variations in wage rates and salaries. For example, one of the justifications for increasing pay with job seniority is that the longer a person performs a particular job, the more skilled he/she becomes in its execution.

Would such a procedure be appropriate for studies of health manpower productivity? Unfortunately, the nature of pricing and price setting in the health sector appear to present insurmountable difficulties. One problem is the difference between fees and actual charges for physician services. Another is the lack of an adequate competitive structure which would insure that the prices of low quality procedures and outputs would fall while high quality prices rise. A third difficulty, primarily in the hospital sector, is that many services are priced at cost, rather than at their relative values to patients. An example might be helpful here.

Suppose we consider the case of a particular hospital-based treatment of an unspecified condition, "Malady X." Let us assume that for some reason the hospital determined that it could provide the same treatment for Malady X with a lower personnel to patient ratio. Now there is clearly no change in output, and there is a decrease in labor input—a clear case of higher productivity. Given the nature of the hospital industry, how would this case appear when an attempt was made to estimate productivity change from available data? The estimate of productivity change would be derived from dividing the estimated value of output by the labor input at the two points in time and comparing them. Labor inputs would be lower, but what of the estimated value of output? The output of the hospital industry is essentially priced at cost. It is clear that the estimate could reflect no change in productivity when the very example was postulated to reflect an unambiguous increase in productivity. The problem, of course, is with the price information in the hospital industry. . . . It should be apparent that lower productivity translates into higher costs. In those cases it is clearly inappropriate to use costs as an approximation of the value of output to derive estimates of productivity changes.[10]

This whole problem is further confounded by the fact that some "profitable" services are frequently overpriced or overcharged in order to cross-subsidize other unprofitable services.

By now the general difficulties associated with measuring and incorporating quality changes should be clear. Even under the best of conditions there is no technique which fully accounts for quality, and in the health sector the measurement problems become all the more severe. One possible exit from this dilemma is through the creation of a Relative Value Scale along the lines of the one used in California. Currently, however, such indices are limited in scope and have yet to be fully validated. Therefore, in reporting the results of previous productivity studies, our implicit assumption will be that quality was held approximately constant over the course of the research. Subjectively, however, each reader may slant the estimates of productivity increases either upwards or downwards depending upon whether he/she believes quality to have risen or declined as a result of the productivity-changing measure. Thus, if one feels that organizing physicians in group practice increases the quality of care because of greater peer monitoring and continuing education, then the *measured* productivity increase will underestimate the true increase.

Although quality measurement is by far the greatest problem associated with analyzing health manpower productivity, there are a number of other caveats which should also be kept in mind. One is that increasing health manpower productivity is only an intermediate goal toward the final objective of improving health levels. Consequently, the paradoxical situation may arise in which policies which increase health may also lead to a decrease in productivity. For example, many have argued that an effective policy for improving health would be an expansion of "preventative" type measures, which may or may not be medically based. One implication of such a policy is that as prevention becomes more and more successful, the average health status of the patient actually seeking a physician's services is likely to decline. Other things equal, one would expect this to lead to a decline in measured productivity. A similar effect might be observed from policies which effectively exclude well patients from entering the medical system.

The relationships between technical change, biomedical research, and medical practice is another example. Much of the recent medical technology has been the kind which postpones death or compensates for the effects of disease, rather than actually curing or preventing disease (Thomas, 1971). Organ transplants, hemodialysis, and the management of coronary heart disease are good examples of this kind of technology. While these techniques may be viewed as "medical miracles," they are also extremely complex and expensive in terms of the amount of resources they require. Whether or not these are the "right" technologies, and whether or not their outcomes justify their expense are questions obviously beyond the scope of this document. However, policies which improve health through such new technology may also lead to a reduction in productivity, as currently measured.

Even where the literature indicates the possible existence of economically feasible productivity gains, we are still faced with the problems of (1) inducing movement to the higher productivity state and (2) insuring that the productivity increases are passed on to consumers in the form of lower costs. The former would generally require a good knowledge of the behavior patterns of the health sector's relevant actors-physicians, patients, ancillary personnel, administrators, etc., and of the interactions between behavior and the system's institutional and technological constraints. The second problem involves the issues of how physicians set their prices, and of their relative tradeoffs between higher incomes and more leisure. Thus, it is conceivable that without the proper guidelines or mechanisms, productivity-increasing measures could lead to greater physician leisure at the same output and income levels.

More mundane than the above consideration, but nonetheless relevant, are problems associated with data scarcity and the relative nescience of health economics research. Probably the germinal work in health economics research was Klarman's *The Economics of Health* which appeared only in 1965. Since then, intensive work has uncovered many important structural and behavioral relationships of the health care sector. However, given the great complexity of the health system relative to the typical kinds of markets studied by economists, it is still far too early for a complete understanding of the complex *interrelationships* between the various parts of the system.

Empirical research has been hampered by the nonexistence (or at least the nonusability) of many kinds of data, especially, for example, information on consumer utilization of medical services, the employment patterns of nonnurse ancillaries, and physician income and practice techniques. In a similar way research on multispecialty group practice has been limited by the relative newness of this form of organization, particularly of large size groups. The largest group practice plan (Kaiser-Permanente) has so far refused to open its data to outside researchers. Confidentiality has also proved to be a significant barrier to research on physician behavior. Data from the AMA and *Medical Economics* has generally not been available to outside researchers. It is only in the last two years that economics researchers have had access to the AMA's Periodic Survey of Physicians. (Both projects are funded by BHSR, and are still in progress.[11]) Consequently, many of the conclusions below must be based on first cuts at a very complex system. Where empirical knowledge is lacking, theoretical considerations will be brought to bear. One must keep in mind, however, that many of these have not yet been satisfactorily tested.

Changes in Productivity

Once a definition has been determined, changes in productivity can occur in several ways. In particular, an increase in productivity will be said to have taken place if (1) the quantity of output increases for a given level of input(s), or (2) the quantity of input(s) required to produce a given quantity of output decreases.[12] It should be noted that these are tautological descriptions of productivity change derived from the definition of productivity as "output per unit of input," and not sources or causes of productivity changes. The important point is that when identifying a change in productivity all inputs but one should implicitly be held constant.[13] If two or more factors change simultaneously, the effect on productivity is likely to be ambiguous. Thus, while it is true that almost any increase in the quantity of inputs will also increase output, it is not necessarily true that all such changes are productivity improving. This is the distinction underlying the difference between technical feasibility and economic feasibility (to be explained in greater detail below) in evaluating proposed productivity-increasing alternatives.

Plan of the Chapter

The following section will briefly summarize past sources and potential future sources of productivity growth, relying on the frame of reference developed above. We will then summarize the state-of-the-art as it pertains to each of the potential sources of future productivity growth. As stated above, the main emphasis will be on physician productivity, although issues relevant to allied health manpower will also be mentioned. Following the statement-of-knowledge summaries, the last section of Chapter 7 will be devoted to suggesting areas where future research is needed; we will also derive and discuss policy implications which follow from consideration of the available pertinent knowledge about health manpower productivity.

Potential Sources of Productivity Growth

Sources of Productivity Growth in the Past

It is possible to attribute a fairly large portion of the growth in postwar physician productivity to two general sources. Since the 1930s there has been a drastic reallocation of physician's time from house calls to office and hospital visits and to telephone consultations. In 1930 home visits comprised 45 percent of all outpatient visits; in 1965 they were only 4 percent of the total (Reinhardt, 1970, p. 13). Since the average house call takes up to three times as much physician time as an office visit, it is apparent that this substitution of patient for physician effort has resulted in substantial time saving for the physician. It is also apparent that this particular source of productivity growth is unlikely to contribute much in the future to productivity increases.

The second major source of productivity growth can be traced to advances in biomedical knowledge and techniques, and in the development of antibiotics

(Fuchs and Kramer, 1972, pp. 13-14); see Table 7-1. During the late 1940s and early 1950s many drugs were introduced which were highly effective against influenza, pneumonia, tuberculosis, and other infectious diseases which had large impacts on morbidity and mortality. These drugs included penicillin (discovered in 1928 but not widely diffused until the 1940s), streptomycin, chlortetracycline, (the first broad spectrum antibiotic) in 1949, tetracycline in 1953, and para-amino-salicyclic acid and isoniazid for tuberculosis treatment. Since 1956, however, the tenor of technological development has changed. New advances have typically been of the kind which have only a small impact on general health and, at the same time, are highly resource intensive. Chemotherapy and radiation therapy in cancer treatment, hemodialysis, open heart surgery, and organ transplants are examples of this trend.

There has also been a fairly steady substitution of ancillaries for physicians over the period. For example, Weiss found that if the 1950 input coefficients for health manpower had been maintained to produce the 1960 output of the industry, there would have had to be 46,000 more physicians than were actually practicing in 1960, and far fewer employees in the jobs requiring less intensive medical training (Reinhardt, 1970, p. 11; Weiss, 1966). However, this result does not allow for the effects of the changes in medical technology and in the pattern of physician-patient contacts. Intuitively, it seems that these last two were more likely to have made the largest contribution to productivity increases.

Input Substitution

It should be apparent from the general definition of productivity that one way to increase physician productivity in particular, and health manpower productiv-

Table 7-1
Rates of Change of Death Rates and Hospital Use, 1948-1968

	(Percent per Annum Continuously Compounded)			
	1948-56[a]	1956-66	1966-68	1948-68[a]
Death rate, all causes	−0.7 (0.2)	0.0 (0.1)	n.a.	−0.1 (0.1)
Death rate, all causes except heart disease and cancer	−2.0 (0.3)	−0.2 (0.2)	n.a.	−0.6 (0.1)
Average length of hospital stay (days)[b]	−1.3 (0.2)	0.2 (0.1)	3.1 (1.1)	−0.2 (0.1)
Hospital days per 100 persons[b]	0.4 (0.2)	1.7 (0.1)	2.8 (0.9)	1.3 (0.1)

Note: Standard errors of rates of change are shown in parentheses.
[a]Periods shown for death rates are 1949-56 and 1949-67.
[b]Nonfederal short-term general hospitals.
Source: Fuchs and Kramer (1972), p. 14.

ity in general, is through a more effective utilization of the production function inputs. One obvious direction of change is the substitution of less expensive units of health manpower (physician assistants, MEDEX, midwives, hygienists, etc.) for the more expensive types of manpower, especially physicians and dentists. Another type of substitution is the replacement of manpower inputs by capital equipment. Increased use of the computer in both medical records and the less traditional areas of diagnosis, treatment, and patient monitoring come to mind. Inpatient and outpatient care facilities might also be designed so as to reduce staff requirements for given levels of output.

The general issues involved in the analysis of input substitution are whether technical possibilities for substitution exist, and, if they do, are they economically feasible? Technical feasibility implies only that physically measured output increases per unit of input. Economic feasibility requires, on the other hand, that the value of the increased output exceeds the cost of implementing and maintaining the proposed substitution. For example, installation of a computer monitoring system may indeed reduce, say, nurse requirements per intensive care unit. However, if the cost of the computer system and its required programming and maintenance exceeds the salaries of the reduced nurse requirement, then this bit of capital substitution is not economically feasible. Further, even if profitable opportunities for input substitution do exist, we must ask if present incentives will induce the desired changes. Finally, we must consider whether there are mechanisms which insure that the potential productivity gains will be passed on to the consumer, rather than accrue entirely to the physician?

A second general type of input substitution would use the patient as a more active member of the health team. Possibilities for involving the patient in diagnosis, treatment, and management of his illness will be examined.

Organizational Changes

In addition to possibilities for altering the proportions in which production function inputs are combined, we will also examine the effects of changing the institutional setting of medical care production. The most visible suggestion along these lines has been to organize physicians in group practices rather than in the more traditional solo practices. Evidence concerning possible productivity gains in both single- and multi-specialty groups will be presented.

Comparison of the effects of different types of reimbursement schemes may also be examined under the heading of organizational changes. Traditionally, physicians have been paid on fee-for-service basis, but it has been argued that this method of reimbursement has incentives for "overdoctoring patients (Ginzberg, 1966; p. 86). Presumably, physicians who are either salaried or paid on a capitation basis will have incentives to (1) economize on their own input for given output levels, and (2) increase output for a given level of physician input, respectively. These alternative types of reimbursement schemes are frequently mentioned in conjunction with the formation of group practices. Therefore, where appropriate, the two will be analyzed together.

Part of the institutional structure within which medical practices are carried out is defined in terms of state laws, statutes, and other legal regulations. Most prominent among these are licensure conditions for both physician and other health personnel. The effects of licensure on productivity will thus also be examined in this section.

Changes in the Quality and Distribution of Health Manpower

For a given combination of outputs and inputs we would expect, in general, that an increase in the quality of the manpower inputs would increase productivity. As in the discussion of the quality of medical care, the notion of manpower quality is also very vague. There is no unambiguous definition, measurement is difficult, and we do not have very good notions of how changes in quality came about. Three possible approaches are through more careful selection of health professionals, alterations in the educational structure, and closer monitoring of practicing physicians.

It is also fairly well known that there are variations in physician productivity (and presumably in that of other health manpower as well) across medical specialties and over geographic areas. Existing evidence regarding the "productivity spread" will be examined, as will be possible behavioral and structural barriers to specialty and/or location reallocation.

Technical Change

The final source of potential productivity growth to be considered is shifts in the production function itself. In discussing technical change, it will be useful to distinguish between two general ways in which technology effects the production function and manpower productivity. One may be called *process innovation*. This refers to an alteration in the nature of the relationship between inputs and outputs. The other is *product innovation*, which may be thought of as the development of new outputs and inputs.

As will become apparent, there will be some overlap with the section dealing with organizational changes and with capital substitution, since these are frequently the mechanisms which embody new processes or products. Emphasis in this section, however, will be on the relationship between new technology and productivity, and on the way new technologies are developed and diffused.

Input Substitution

Ancillary Personnel

The relevant questions regarding the increased utilization of ancillary personnel are (1) do technical opportunities for input substitution exist, and, if they do, are they economically feasible; (2) will these opportunities be adopted; and (3) who appropriates the gains from increased productivity? In attempting to investigate these questions, production function techniques have been used by Reinhardt (1972), Reinhardt and Yett (1971), Kehrer and Zaretsky (1972), Bailey (1968), and Kimball and Lorant (1972); activity analysis has been used by Golladay, Smith, and Miller (1971), and much less structured utilization surveys have been used by Yankauer, Connelly, and Feldman (1970), Riddick et al. (1971).

Reinhardt (1972) and Reinhardt and Yett (1970) used cross-section data from *Medical Economics* surveys in 1965 and 1967 to estimate a production function for solo physicians (obstetrics, gynecology, and internal medicine) in private practice. Included as inputs were measures of registered nurses per physician, technicians per physician, and office aides per physician. Reinhardt (1972, p. 61) estimated that the marginal productivity of an auxiliary tended to increase up to the level of about one aide per physician, diminishing thereafter, and becoming negative at a level between 5.0 and 5.5 aides per physician. The general results of these two studies were that at prevailing wages, the average solo practitioner could profitably employ almost twice as many ancillary personnel as are currently being used, i.e., from 1.9 to 4 aides per physician (Reinhardt and Yett, 1971, p. 27). This would result in approximately a 25 percent increase in the number of total patient visits per week per physician. Kehrer and Zaretsky (1972), using different data and different functional specifications,[14] found results surprisingly similar to Reinhardt's. They concluded that in general a doubling of allied health personnel input would increase total patient visits per physician by 20 to 25 percent (p. 95). The marginal product curves for ancillaries tended to become negative at generally higher levels of aids per physician than in Reinhardt's work, and there were wide variations across medical specialties. Their estimates implied that internal medicine and general practice appeared most capable of absorbing additional ancillaries. This is consistent with the general feeling that the less esoteric the specialty, the greater the opportunities for delegating tasks to paramedicals. Finally, Kimbell and Lorant (1972) also used AMA data [Seventh Periodic Survey of Physicians (1972)] to estimate production functions for private practitioners. Although their actual estimates differ somewhat from previous work, their general conclusions are highly consistent with the results of previous studies. Table 7-2 illustrates some of these results.

Table 7-2
Production Functions for Private Practitioners

A. Estimated Effect of Physician Hours and of Aides on the Rate of Physician Output (Solo General Practitioners)

Number of Physician Hours per Week	Number of Aides per Physician						
	0	0.5	1	2	3	4	5
Total practice hours	Total Patient Visits per Week[a]						
40	85	96	107	128	146	159	165
60	123	139	155	185	212	230	239
Office hours	Office Visits per Week[b]						
25	73	85	99	122	142	154	156
35	91	107	122	153	178	193	196
Total practice hours	Patient Billings per Year[c]						
40	28.1	32.1	36.1	43.9	50.8	55.7	58.1
60	36.0	41.1	46.2	56.3	65.0	71.4	74.4

B. Number of Allied Health Personnel at Which Their Marginal Product Is at a Maximum and Is Equal to Zero (Four Primary Care Specialty Groups)

Specialty Group	Number of AHPs at Max. MP	Number of AHPs at Zero MP
General Practice	4.8	19.4
Internal Medicine	13.2	26.0
Obstetrics-Gynecology	2.0	8.2
Pediatrics	0.6	6.9

[a]Sample averages of total visits, total practice hours and aides per physician for solo GPs were 183, 60 and 1.81, respectively.

[b]Sample averages of office visits and office hours were about 36 and 150, respectively.

[c]Annual patient billings, in thousands of dollars, based on 1965 income data. The sample average for that year was $55.0.

Sources: Reinhardt (1972), p. 63; Kehrer and Zaretsky (1972), p. 87.

Acitivity analysis was used by Golladay, Miller, and Smith (1971, 1972), to develop a *normative* model of how a primary care practice *should* be organized. The procedure consisted of enumerating 263 tasks in eight major categories of activity which fully described a primary care practice. In order to determine the frequency with which tasks were delegated, five medical school students acted as observers in a sample of primary care practice in Wisconsin, Vermont, and North Carolina over two-week periods. In the actual analysis, subsets of tasks were aggregated to form medical services.

Solution of their model provides the minimum labor cost and input mix for any given level of output. Their results were predicated on the assumptions that the physician devotes 28 hours a week on direct patient care, that all tasks not classified as being part of some medical service can be delegated to the same extent as included tasks, and that output is at a level such that further delegation of tasks is not possible. Given these assumptions, they find that the productivity of the individual physician could be increased by 74 percent (from 147 visits to 265 visits) by using a Physician's Assistant (Golladay, Smith, and Miller, 1971, p. 20). It should be emphasized, however, that these are *potential* gains which depend crucially on the above assumptions and the additional implicit assumption that physicians are efficient in organizing their practices. In terms of Physician's Assistants, it is also interesting to note that in another study, Scheffler and Stinson (1972) estimated the mean starting salary of a PA to be $10,501 while the possible gain to the physician is two to three times as much.

Surveys of ancillary utilization patterns and the distribution of tasks delegated by pediatricians were undertaken by Yankauer, Connelly, and Feldman (1970a) and Riddick et al. (1971). While not addressing themselves directly to potential productivity gains, they reveal some interesting facts. Yankauer, Connelly, and Feldman found that pediatricians in the Northeast delegate less frequently than physicians in the West, and also that the ratio of ancillaries to physicians is lower in the Northeast than the West (1970a, p. 527). As for task delegation, "The patient care tasks most frequently delegated are those which reflect the most urgent pressures of practice (telephone calls) or those most easily routinized (interpretation of instructions and routine history taking). The tasks least frequently delegated are those which involve clinical judgment or a more intimate patient-caretaker relationship" (p. 535). (See Table 7-3.)

One possible explanation of the observed regional differences in personnel per physician and the distribution of task delegation is that physicians are more likely to have ancillaries and delegate tasks the greater the degree of *excess* demand. (Note that this refers to the *difference* between the quantities of services demanded and supplied, not the absolute level of demand.) One would expect that pressures upon a physician's time would be greatest under these conditions, and further, that the average degree of necessity or complexity of the cases treated by the doctor himself would be higher. Rafferty (1971) has found a similar relationship between demand pressures and case-mix for hospital admissions. Riddick (1971) also found an inverse correlation between the physician-population ratio (a very rough index of relative degrees of excess demand) and both the number of ancillary personnel employed and the degree to which the physician delegates aspects of the practice to assistants.

The evidence presented above suggests several things. First, ancillary marginal productivity is probably highest in areas characterized as having relative shortages of physicians. Secondly, primary care practices appear to have the greatest potential for increasing productivity through greater employment of allied health personnel. Thirdly, physicians are more likely to utilize ancillaries the greater the demands on their time.

Table 7-3

Performance and Delegation of Office, Technical, Laboratory, and Clerical Tasks as Reported by Pediatric Practitioners, U.S.A.

Task	MD	RN	LBP	HA	LT	Sec.	Comb.	ND
				% of 4,208 in Each Category Performed by[a]				

Task	MD	RN	LBP	HA	LT	Sec.	Comb.	ND
Technical Tasks								
Weighing	13	35	10	24	1	7	10	–
Body measurement	23	32	9	21	1	5	8	1
Vision screening	23	29	8	15	2	4	8	10
Hearing screening	38	17	5	8	2	2	5	21
Immunization	41	39	7	6	1	–	5	–
Parent. drugs	47	35	6	4	1	–	4	2
B.P. (older)	66	21	4	4	–	–	3	1
Develop. screening	68	4	1	2	–	–	1	21
B.P. (infant)	76	5	1	1	–	–	1	14
Laboratory Tasks								
Blood count/smear	13	6	1	5	31	1	2	39
Urinalysis	21	16	4	11	30	3	3	10
Hemoglobin	21	13	3	8	30	1	3	19
Venous blood	49	2	–	1	19	–	–	25
Throat culture	59	10	2	3	7	–	3	14
Clerical Tasks								
Inventory/supply	6	35	7	18	2	21	9	1
Insurance forms	13	9	2	11	1	54	8	1
Growth charting	44	16	4	9	1	5	4	15

Note: MA = "Medical Assistant"; LT = laboratory technician; Sec. = secretary; Comb. = combination of two or more health workers (80 percent of combinations include RN); ND = not done in pediatric office.

[a]Percentages are rounded to nearest whole number. Nonresponse rates are not shown but were less than 3 percent for any single task category.

Source: Yankauer, Connelly, and Feldman (1970a), p. 532.

There appear to be, therefore, substantial gains in physician productivity available through increased ancillary utilization. Tables 7-4 and 7-5 indicate the extent to which physicians themselves feel that task delegation could be increased. The question then is why haven't physicians availed themselves of these opportunities?

Current work at the Human Resources Research Center has suggested several theoretical reasons why physicians might not hire as many ancillaries as technically suggested (1972c). These are (1) quality deterioration and a resultant weakening of the doctor-patient relationship, (2) patient resistance, (3) loss of

Table 7-4

Office Patient Care Tasks According to Present Performance and Opinion about Their Delegation

Tasks	Percentage of Total Pediatricians[a]		
	Favoring Delegation (1)	Now Delegating (2)	(1) (2)
Information/childcare	95	26	3.65
Information/immunization	91	45	2.02
Interpret instruction	85	30	2.83
Telephone/childcare	78	48	1.62
Family social history	75	41	1.83
Interval history/well child	65	16	4.06
Past medical history	64	33	1.94
Advice/feeding-development	63	22	2.87
Telephone/minor medical advice	58	55	1.06
Advice/minor medical	52	30	1.73
Interval/history sick child	45	16	2.81
Advice/school child	40	6	6.07
Present illness history	39	22	1.77
Exam/well child	25	5	5.00
Exam/sick child	20	12	1.67

[a]Percentages are only approximations.

Source: Adapted from Figure 14 in Yankauer, Connelly, and Feldman (1970a), p. 540.

physician-patient personal relationship, (4) managerial disutilities, (5) disutilities from too large a practice, (6) increased likelihood of malpractice suits and higher malpractice insurance rates, (7) costs of on-the-job training, (8) space limitations, and (9) licensure limits on what tasks ancillaries are legally qualified to perform. Investigation of most of these is difficult with existing data. However, the HRRC will attempt to investigate the relative importance of patient resistance, disutilities associated with a large practice, managerial disutilities, malpractice insurance, and space limitations.

As part of this effort, Intriligator and Kehrer (1972, p. 29) have developed a simultaneous equations model attempting to explain the employment of ancillary personnel in physicians' offices. The data were from the AMA's Seventh Periodic Survey of Physicians. While still in a preliminary stage of development, the early results indicate that the size of malpractice insurance premiums did not have a significant impact upon physicians' decisions regarding ancillaries. This conclusion was also reached by the President's Commission on Malpractice (1973, p. 48). As the authors point out, however, insurance premiums may not fully capture the threat or fear of malpractice suits.

Table 7-5

Extent of Present Delegation to Allied Health Workers and Extent to Which Internists Believe Delegation Should be Made

	Percent of Offices		
	Now Delegating Specified Tasks United States (1)	Believe Could and Should Be Delegated United States (2)	(2) (1)
Laboratory and Related Tasks			
Obtain and mount electro-cardiogram tracings	93.6	–	–
Obtain venous blood samples for lab	72.2	93.8	1.29
Procure urine sample for lab	96.2	–	–
Perform urinalysis (glucose, protein)	93.8	97.3	1.03
Prepare urine for microanalysis	91.5	97.4	1.06
Determine hemoglobin	31.1	97.6	1.07
Determine hematrocrit	92.8	97.6	1.05
Perform blood cell counts smears or both	90.9	97.1	1.07
Perform pulmonary function studies	58.5	88.8	1.52
Perform Master's two-step exercise test			
Perform skin tests [allergic, fungi, tuberculosis (TBc)]	46.7	76.9	1.65
Therapy			
Administer immunizations	63.2	89.7	1.42
Administer medications intramuscularly	60.5	90.2	1.49
Administer medications intravenously	11.8	41.8	3.54
Perform ear irrigations	25.8	67.4	2.61
Remove sutures	18.0	69.3	3.85
Give diet instruction for obesity, diabetes, etc.	19.7	70.6	3.58
Clerical and Office Tasks			
Fill out insurance forms	85.6	–	–
Do billing	98.4	–	–
Order refills of prescriptions with your authorization	84.0	93.4	.99

Table 7-5 (cont.)

	Percent of Offices		
	Now Delegating Specified Tasks United States (1)	Believe Could and Should Be Delegated United States (2)	(2) (1)
Schedule appointments for X-ray and lab work	94.0	97.2	1.04
Schedule admissions to hospital	66.4	87.0	1.31
Schedule appointments on referral cases without conferring with you	75.7	84.0	1.11
Schedule appointments on referral cases after conferring with you	91.6	96.4	1.05
Type progress notes on chart	70.3	–	–
Physical Examination Tasks			
Obtain height and weight	80.5		
Take blood pressure on initial visit	17.0	–	–
Take blood pressure in following hypertensive patient	21.1	–	–
Take temperature	76.5	–	–
Administer screening tests for hearing	47.4	93.0	1.96
Administer screening tests for vision	69.2	93.0	1.36
Perform tonometry	15.2	50.9	3.35
Perform proctoscopic examination	1.1	9.1	8.27
Perform pelvic examination and do pap smear	0.8	6.3	7.87
Perform pap smear only	3.1	33.7	10.87
History and Patient Contact Tasks			
Take and record routine elements of history (family, operations, injuries, etc.)	12.7	60.3	4.75
Take and record history of present illness	4.4	28.1	6.39
Take and record elements of systemic review	5.1	37.4	7.33
Provide telephone advice on routine medical questions	43.2	60.6	1.40

Table 7-5 (cont.)

	Now Delegating Specified Tasks United States (1)	Percent of Offices Believe Could and Should Be Delegated United States (2)	(2) (1)
Provide (a) telephone advice on routine minor medical problems and (b) schedule patient for examination at office if she thinks it necessary	75.5	(a) 66.7 (b) 76.6	(a) 0.88 (b) 1.01
Visit nursing homes for routine medical rechecks	2.5	46.6	17.12
Visit patients' homes to determine necessity of physicians' exam at home	15.2	64.9	4.27

Source: Riddick (1971), p. 926.

Another point which may be relevant to the greater use of Physician's Assistants is that current legislative, reimbursement, and credentialing procedures are tending to force PAs into areas where there are physicians with practices large enough for the financial justification of the employment of an assistant.[15]

... This produces a situation in which the assistant will find himself forced into physicians' offices and areas in which his contribution to those now receiving inadequate care, or no care at all, will be minimal. Generally, this will not help better utilize the talents of the physician, nor will it enhance the distribution of physicians in areas that are most in need of them. The result will be that those now in need of medical care, such as the rural and urban poor and the aged, will continue to be so. The assistant must be given more latitude and the physician less legal responsibility if the assistant is to be able to perform more than glorified nursing duties.[16]

The final concern is with whether or not potential productivity gains, if realized, would be passed on to consumers in the form of lower costs. Evidence here is very skimpy. Only Bailey's work (1968), a study of a number of San Francisco area internists over a two year period, is indirectly relevant. He found that office visits per physician did not increase with group size, but there was an increase in the share of gross billings generated by fees from ancillary services (p. 271). This suggests that the physicians observed substituted increased leisure for the gains in productivity. While one would not want to generalize from this one case, it does indicate that some thought should be paid to mechanisms for passing on productivity gains.

Capital Substitution

Possibilities for increasing health manpower productivity through the substitution of capital for other production function inputs have generally not been explored by economists. There is, however, a fairly large literature developed by engineering and computer oriented specialists. This literature naturally reflects the perspectives and concerns of those groups and, as such, is usually not directly relevant to the framework established in this chapter. The main issue in most cases is whether the new type of capital (or new technology embodied in some type of equipment) increases output or reduces costs per procedure relative to the prior modality. Comparisons of the *full* costs of implementing and maintaining the proposed configuration with the value of the extra output, and implications for health manpower, are frequently not made; that is, the usual objective has been the demonstration of technical rather than economic feasibility. This section summarizes the more relevant pieces of that literature and discusses the postulated productivity gains from capital substitution.

The overwhelming body of this work to date has been concerned with the possibilities for increased use of computer-based practices in health services delivery. Barnett (1968) has identified seven major areas of computer applications in medicine: medical diagnosis, clinical laboratory, screening, patient monitoring, medical records, automated medical history, and hospital information systems. The particular research efforts reported below fall into these categories. Additionally, Waxman and Rockoff (1972) have indicated the possibilities of using communications technologies to overcome barriers created by geographic dispersion and transportation difficulties. Because of large capital costs and frequently high volume requirements, the institutional setting for just about all this research has been either hospital inpatient, or clinic, or outpatient department based ambulatory care. Diffusion of low cost computer terminals or other communications equipment into physicians' offices and/or patients' homes is still only at the conceptual stage of development.

The potential payoffs from increased computerization appear four-fold.

1. By performing many of the routine tasks associated with patient diagnosis and management, computers may reduce the required input of physician, nurse, and other ancillary personnel time. The types of activities currently being explored are reading X-rays, EKGs, and EEGs, analyzing blood, urine, and other lab tests, recording patient histories, and monitoring patients' vital signs.
2. Physician time can also be conserved by means of a more effective triage

function, operating through either a multiphasic screening type mechanism, or computer assisted history taking by paramedical personnel.

3. Institutional operating costs may be lowered because of more efficient auditing, cost accounting, and interdepartmental coordination.

4. Finally, improved assessment and evaluation of services provided and improved information for research and teaching may be possible with the collection of baseline and continuing data on the population treated. While the third and fourth are clearly important to the performance of the medical care delivery system as a whole, the first two are more relevant to this report.

Studies of diagnosis-assisting computer uses have been done by Berkeley Scientific Laboratories (1971) who examined automated clinical laboratory systems, and Elliott (1972) who investigated computer-assisted analysis and interpretation of electrocardiograms. In observing hospitals which have automated their chemistry laboratories, the Berkeley study found a very rapid rate of growth in workload (about 15 percent per year), and that cost per test *ordered* remains approximately the same as in a manual test setting (Waxman and Rockoff, 1972, p. 2). This is in spite of the fact that the cost per automated test is less than half ($0.24 per test as opposed to $0.52 per test at a volume of 250 tests per day) that of a manual test. The difficulty, apparently, is that the automated equipment performs upwards of eight tests per specimen, not all of which were ordered (Berkeley Labs., 1971, pp. 213-14). At very large volumes, significant economies become apparent, e.g., at 2500 tests per day cost is as low as $0.07 per test. Unfortunately, there is no attempt to assess the value to the physician of additional lab tests, nor is it clear that there are any reductions in personnel or in total laboratory costs including the costs of computer support personnel.

Elliott (1972) documents the three-year history of a contract awarded to the Community Electrocardiograph Interpretive Service (CEIS) of Denver, Colorado to determine whether a set of computer programs could be structured into a community-wide operating system capable of providing computer-assisted EKG interpretation in a clinical setting. A total of 20 hospitals in four states with an overall capacity of 2,387 beds participated in the demonstration. Like the automated clinical laboratory tests reported above, cost per EKG diagnosis declines rapidly as output increases, going from $14.06 per EKG at a volume of 60 readings per day to $0.58 per EKG at the maximum volume 1,440 EKGs per day. Average daily volume at CEIS has been 125 per day, but is expected to rise to 165 per day, which represents 11.5 percent of the system's capacity (Elliott, 1972, p. 52). At this volume, cost is estimated to be $5.11 per EKG. If one adds to this the $2.00 cost of obtaining the EKG from the patient, and the electrocardiographer's $5.00 fee for overreading the computer diagnosis, then total cost per EKG at this volume is $12.00 (Elliott, 1972, p. xiv). Although data is not overly reliable, estimates of the cost of nonautomated EKG services in the Denver area range from $8.00 to $15.00 per EKG (Waxman and Rockoff, 1972, p. 2).

On the basis of this study and other studies reviewed in the report, it was determined that the computer interpretation grossly agrees with the electrocardiographer 85 to 90 percent of the time, with the approximate saving of half of his/her time on the average compared to the conventional method of interpreting the EKG (Elliott, 1972, p. 81). However, conversion to a computer system results in a discreet jump of approximately 8 percent in the number of EKGs performed (p. 37). When combined with an overall growth rate of 12 percent in EKGs performed, it is apparent that some of the potential saving in electrocardiographers' time is consumed by increased volume levels. As in the Berkeley Lab study, there is no analysis of the value of the additional number of EKGs compared to total system costs or possible changes in required personnel.

Reiffen and Komaroff (1972 p. 1) are developing a system of

... problem-oriented protocols to guide the efforts of non-physician paramedics in helping manage conditions which account for the most frequent number of patient visits to ambulatory care settings. The protocols direct the collection by the paramedic of a history, physical examination, and laboratory data keyed to the reason for the patient's visit.

An experiment involving a Chronic Disease Protocol was performed by the Diabetes Clinic of the Boston City Hospital from February 1972 through December 1972. A total of 241 visits were divided into a protocol group (165) and a control group (76). Comparisons were then made along several dimensions of an evaluation scheme. Quality of care was measured by examining the blood sugar levels of two groups with homogeneous medical conditions following a visit to the physician alone or to the paramedic-protocol. The difference between the average change, while not statistically significant, did appear to support a trend in favor of protocol visits. Of the patients who kept their appointments with the protocol service, 40 (37 percent) required no further referral to a physician. Finally, on the basis of several criteria, both patient and physician acceptance of protocol use seemed fairly high (Reiffen and Komaroff, 1972, pp. 11-15). A Phase 3 Evaluation is expected to compute the costs of the protocol system, and compare them to the value of physician time saved, and to the value of possible changes in patient time consumed by a clinic visit (door-to-door).

Waxman and Rockoff (1972, p. 3) have reported the results of automated medical history taking in two other settings, the Massachusetts General Hospital Outpatient Clinic and five-person internal medicine group practice in Washington, D.C. In both instances, a physician further annotated the medical history in the patient's presence and saved 20 to 30 minutes for each new patient workup by this process. For the Washington study this could be translated into savings of $17.00 to $25.00 per history (20 to 30 minutes at $50.00 per hour for an internist) which offset computer costs in a *low volume* situation of about $12.00 per history. Studies of multiphasic screening [e.g., Garfield (1970)] appear to show increases in patient throughput and reductions in physician time. However, analyses of costs and the value of saved time are not yet available.

As can be seen from this section, research into possibilities for capital substitution is a fairly new endeavor, with a strong bias towards computer-based technologies. Work concerned with either the more conventional types of capital or the relatively esoteric types of noncomputer hardware is practically nonexistent.[17] The impressionistic evidence regarding the latter, however, seems to indicate that highly sophisticated capital equipment is very expensive and seems to have only a small impact upon morbidity and mortality rates.[18] More work in both of these areas is clearly needed, as are studies dealing more directly with the issue of economic as opposed to technical feasibility of computer-based systems.

Greater Patient Involvement

The chapter by Fredrick Golladay offers a comprehensive review of the very extensive literature dealing with patient involvement in the medical care process; this section therefore only highlights the main issues under that topic.

The literature dealing with the general area of increased patient participation in the health care system is not only extensive in its range, but also fragmentary, in the sense that seldom are more than a small subset of the relevant issues discussed. This is due in part to the lack of any generally agreed upon notions of what patient participation is, where in the health care system increased participation should be applied, and what effect, if any, this would have on health status. Further, the medical and public health disciplinary origin of most of this literature has resulted in very little attention being paid to the issue of cost effectiveness. This, of course, is the primary concern of the review. Therefore, in the summary which follows, patient participation will be taken to mean not only direct involvement in administering medical treatments, but also participation in determining utilization levels, phasing and monitoring therapy, and organizing and executing programs of health maintenance. The term "patient" will be used to include members of the household, as well as the recipient of care. In selecting articles for inclusion, emphasis was placed upon relevance to the issue of cost effectiveness. Finally, the literature was grouped under the five major headings of health maintenance activities (preventive care), compliance with medical treatment, utilization of the health care system, patient self-care and the effects of patient knowledge.

Preventive care has been a major focus of evaluative research in looking at the usefulness of periodic examinations, Franco et al. (1961), and Wade et al., (1962), both found a considerable amount of undetected disabling diseases. It was not shown, however, that early diagnosis increased treatment effectiveness (David, 1961). Grinaldi (1965), on the other hand, in an analysis of matched groups found that the medical care costs for the control group exceeded those of the experimental group by more than the cost of the periodic examination. In the area of preventing communicable diseases, the value of innoculations is accepted. The issue here is how to induce people to participate in innoculation programs (Golladay, 1973, p. 8). Similarly, the efficacy of early diagnosis of cancer, cardiovascular disease, tuberculosis, and dental disease implies productivity gains from identifying risk factors and signs, and encouraging self-diagnosis.

Interest in the area of patient compliance with medical regimen has been predicated on the assumption that noncompliance erodes the effectiveness of the health care system. One study of elderly ambulatory patients with chemotherapy programs found that more than sixty percent were noncompliant in one way or another (Curtis, 1961; Schwartz et al., 1962). The impact of noncompliance upon treatment efficacy was not investigated, however. In general a good deal of the descriptive literature has focused upon self concept, role definition, and fear of activity loss as factors affecting compliance. The state of the literature is summarized by Simonds (1966):

We are only beginning to understand the problem of patient compliance with medical regimens and some of the related motivational factors. We know that the beliefs the individual holds . . . are strong influencers of action. We know from the work of several social psychologists that beliefs about the medical condition itself and the effectiveness of available courses of preventive or therapeutic actions are significant variables. These beliefs differ between men as contrasted with women; among young people as contrasted with older people; and among people who have different diseases or feel they might get different diseases . . . Available research suggests only that these beliefs tend to be associated with actions reported by the patient. Whether they are causative influencers and, even more important, whether they can be effectively manipulated in the form of educational messages to influence behavior is still largely unknown.

A third focal point of research has been the decision to seek medical care, with particular emphasis upon explaining delays in seeking care. This literature, however, seldom deals with the questions of the appropriateness of intervention or of its optimal timing. Mechanic (1966), Blackwell (1962), and others have examined the willingness of prospective patients to adopt a *sick role*.[19] This implicitly assumes that the appropriate posture for the sick is dependency, and that early treatment is optimal. Other research has found that psychological problems were less readily presented, that ethnicity affected utilization, and that attitudes toward authority and previous experiences with physicians influenced willingness to seek help.

Opportunities for patient self-care would seem to be greatest for chronic diseases which require continuous management, e.g., diabetes, chronic heart diseases, and tuberculosis. Self-care programs for diabetes are the most wide-spread at this time (Ulrich and Kelley, 1972). In a study of an education program for heart patients the experimental group required approximately one-third as many hospital admissions, one-fourth as many days of hospital care, and experienced less than half as many readmissions as the control group (Rosenberg, 1971). Another program at the University of Kentucky Medical Center utilizes children's parents for a good part of inpatient care. In addition to the evident psychological benefits, the cost of hospitalization was reduced approximately 40 percent, and direct personnel costs were reduced from $10.31 per day to $3.81 (James and Wheeler, 1969).

Finally, research examining the extent of patient knowledge indicates that even for common and highly publicized problems, public beliefs and attitudes are inconsistent with either a preventive mode of care or early detection (Golladay, 1973, pp. 16-18). It is not clear, however, if one can expect desirable changes in patient behavior to result from increases or improvements in patient knowledge.

Assuming that one wished to increase patient knowledge, the next relevant question would be what type of educational strategy should be employed. Two distinct traditions have emerged: one emphasizes formal educational programs, and the other advocates information instruction in parallel with professional care.

Studies of formal instruction have reviewed techniques such as printed pamphlets, films, television and group methods, and in-hospital educational programs for patient groups (Golladay, 1973, pp. 18-21). The major problems appear to be motivating learning, determining readiness for instruction, and adapting curricula to the diversity of patient situations.

More appealing approaches emphasize individualization and informal instruction (Golladay, 1973, pp. 22-23). The nursing profession in particular has vigorously advocated this approach. The advantages of integrating treatment and teaching include, in addition to individualization, opportunities to exploit the motivation to learn which frequently accompanies a problem and economics in the use of staff.

Organizational Changes

Group Practice and Other Practice Modes

Comparisons of solo medical practice with group practice are usually concerned with two questions. Are physicians more productive in a group practice setting, and are there economies of scale inherent in the technology of group practice? These issues have been dealt with in detail in chapters by Richard Scheffler and Frank Sloan. While the questions appear superficially similar, there are important conceptual differences between them.

Returning to the framework presented earlier[20] let

$$S = f(L_1, \ldots, L_n, K_1, \ldots, K_n) \tag{7.6}$$

be the production function for a solo practice firm, and

$$G = g(L_1, \ldots, L_n, K_1, \ldots, K_n) \tag{7.7}$$

be the group practice function. Different production functions are appropriate if we believe the production processes to be qualitatively different between the two practice forms.

Focusing on physicians, the productivity question is, "If a number of doctors, D, are available, can more output be obtained by having them practice in one or more groups or by installing them in D solo practices?" Letting each solo practice produce an output S_i, the productivity issue is the direction of the inequality.

$$\frac{G}{D} \underset{<}{\overset{\geq}{}} \sum_{i=1}^{D} \frac{S_i}{D} . \tag{7.8}$$

Productivity of all manpower inputs (or any combination of them) can be compared only if the inputs can be combined into some index, M. Then the proper comparison is given by

$$\frac{G}{M_G} \underset{>}{\overset{\leq}{}} \sum_{i=1}^{D} \frac{\dfrac{S_i}{D}}{\sum\limits_{i=1}^{D} M_i} \tag{7.9}$$

where M_i is the index of inputs for the ith solo practice.

Economies of scale, on the other hand, implies the following question. "If we keep the production processes unchanged, what happens to output as *all* inputs are changed in the same proportion?" We know that multiplying each input by some constant amount, n, will increase output (except in the unlikely case where all inputs have reached zero marginal productivity), i.e.,

$$mG = g(nL_1, \ldots, nLj, nK_1, \ldots, nK_m). \tag{7.10}$$

If $m = n$, then output increases in the same proportion and the production function is said to exhibit constant returns to scale, $m < n$ implies decreasing returns to scale, and $m > n$ implies increasing returns. The nature of returns to scale is important to the determination of the optimum size physician practice. It should be obvious, however, that the question of economies of scale is not relevant to solo practice.

One could also seek to identify the optimum size practice by looking for the minimum point of the average total cost function. Under certain conditions this is identical to using the production function technique for determining optimum scale (Shephard, 1970).

A conceptual difficulty in the literature on productivity and economies of scale in medical practices is obviously that data on solo and group practices cannot be simultaneously used to study both theoretical constructs. Either we believe solo and group practices have the same production function and we examine economies of scale, or we believe they have different production functions and we look at productivity differences between types of practice and economies of scale *within* group practices. This same dilemma arises in comparisons of single- and multi-specialty groups.

Discussions of group practice, particularly multispecialty groups, are frequently tied in with prepayment schemes. While the nature of the reimbursement mechanism is likely to have an effect on physician behavior and productivity, it is nonetheless conceptually distinct from the mode of organization. Fee-for-service is not incompatible with group practice, nor is capitation or prepayment incompatible with solo practice. Therefore, the review of the relationship between productivity and physician reimbursement will be treated separately.

Recognizing these difficulties, Reinhardt (1972) estimated a production function for two physician specialties, obstetricians-gynecologists and internists. His specific assumption was that solo and single-specialty group practices employ the same production function, but at different scales. The data were from 1965 and 1967 surveys conducted by Medical Economics, Inc. His estimates "suggest that, at given levels of practice inputs, physicians in (single-specialty) groups tend to generate between 4.5 and 5.1 percent more patient visits and 5.6 percent more patient billings than do their colleagues in solo practice (p. 60).

Kovner (1968) attempted to use the production function method to measure productivity increases as a function of the size of prepaid group practices. His data was observation of seven outpatient services (office visits, specific diagnostic services, therapeutic services, surgical services, radiological services, laboratory services, and all other) at seven Kaiser Foundation Clinics in Los Angeles. Unfortunately, he did not differentiate these services by diagnostic categories. Further, lack of variation in many of his observations resulted in only seven independent pieces of data. Given these reservations, his results imply increasing returns to scale in prepaid groups as the size of the group increases.

Kimbell and Lorant (1972), also interested in economies of scale, used 990 observations on group practices from a recent AMA Survey of Medical Groups to estimate a production function of the Cobb-Douglas form. Their preliminary estimates indicate that economies of scale are either constant or generally decreasing over the range of firms included in their estimates (from 3 to 100 physicians). Their data, however, included both single and multispecialty groups in the same sample.

Bailey (1968, 1970), attempted to measure economies of scale by comparing rates of office visits for a sample of internists in the San Francisco area during April 1967. Using a visits per physician hour measure of productivity, he found no consistent evidence of economies of scale. Three-man groups appeared the most productive, while four- to five-man groups were least productive. Within the private practice set, the relationship between practice size and visits is nonmonotonic. His data indicated that average internist hours decline as a function of group size (although two-man partners have longer work weeks than solo practitioners). However, income per physician is higher in the larger practices because, he claims, these physicians provide extra ancillary services under one roof, and substitute the revenue from these services for revenues from direct patient care. Furthermore, the ratio of paramedical help to physicians rose as group size increased, while physician productivity was actually smaller and total production per physician remained the same. This also suggests that ancillary time is substituted for physician time. Unfortunately, Bailey's sample size is small, no standard deviations are given, and the method of compensation for the clinic physicians is not specified (thus one cannot disentangle a reimbursement effect from a size effect). Table 7-6 summarizes Bailey's findings.

Newhouse (1973) agrees with Bailey that economies of scale may be present, but they are not likely to be realized. Unlike Bailey, however, he argues that as group size increases, the individual physician's incentives to be efficient diminish because his/her decisions are not likely to have as large an impact upon personal income as they would in smaller groups. Bailey argues, in effect, that the productivity gains are appropriated by the physicians. Newhouse estimated an average cost function (for several types of costs) over a sample of eleven solo, five two-men, one three-man, and two five-man practices. More specifically,

Table 7-6
Bailey's Findings

	Solo	2-Man	3-Man	4 to 5-Man	Clinics
Average M.D. hours[a]	218	222	197	200	197
Paramedical hours/[b] physician hours	0.86	0.82	1.14	1.35	2.53
Weighted office[c] visits/physician	286	278	291	243	286
Weighted office[d] visits/physician hours	1.31	1.25	1.48	1.22	1.45

[a]Bailey (1970), Table 3, p. 270.
[b]Ibid.
[c]Ibid., Table 2.
[d]Computed by dividing visits by hours.
Source: Berki (1972), p. 18.

economies appeared to be present in such nonmedical areas as office salary costs, medical record costs, appointment costs, billing costs, and rent costs. However, since the groups in his sample were either cost or revenue sharing, he argues that there is a disincentive to individual physicians to either keep their costs down or their work efforts high. These so-called X-inefficiencies more than outweigh potential savings in other areas. Newhouse's results, however, are subject to criticism. First, like Kovner, he uses an extremely small sample, which gives rise to inexact estimates. Second, he doesn't distinguish single from multispecialty groups, but merely uses a zero-one dummy variable to differentiate solo from group practices.

Data from the Yankauer et al. (1970b) study of pediatricians is also useful in examining the relationship between practice size and productivity. Size of group, number of aides per pediatrician, hours, and visits are given in Table 7-7, which reveals a pattern similar to Bailey's. Even though the pediatrician-aide ratio is generally higher for the three-, four-, and five-man group than for the two-man partnership, pediatricians in the two-man partnership (with the exception of the two workers-RN absent category), have approximately the same rates of office visits. Like Bailey, the authors are not explicit about cost- and revenue-sharing arrangements.

Berki (1972) has reworked the Yankauer, et al. data so as to highlight the relationships between practice size and productivity. (See Table 7-8).

Holding the number of ancillaries constant, visits per MD appear to decline for practices with three to five or more ancillaries. Holding the number of physicians fixed, the marginal productivity of an additional ancillary seems to be positive for one- and three-physician practices, and nonmonotonic for two-man practices.

Hughes et al. (1972, 1973) have performed two case studies of surgical practices. The first investigated 19 general surgeons in fee-for-service community practice, and the second examined seven general surgeons comprising the surgical staff of a prepaid group practice with 158,000 enrollees. Using the California Relative Value Scale to translate operations of varying complexity into hernia equivalent (HE) units (One HE is defined as the amount of work involved in the operative and pre- and post-operative care of a patient undergoing an adult unilateral inguinal herniorraphy), they calculated mean and median operative workloads three times larger than the fee-for-service community surgeons, 9.9 and 3.1 HEs per week, respectively. Median complexity was approximately 1.0 HE, and was similar in both studies. While these results are highly provocative, they are somewhat difficult to interpret. For example, the higher productivity of the group surgeons may be due to (1) the prepayment mechanism, which in theory provides incentives to be economically efficient in the production of services (2) economies of scale inherent in the group practice mode (3) extremes of efficient or inefficient production *behavior* on the part of either of the two study groups, or (4) some combination of the above factors.

Table 7-7
Pediatricians

Type of Practice	Direct Hours Worked (in Office Only)	Visits (in Office Only)	
Solo			
1 worker (RN absent)	31.0	81.5	(2.60)
2 workers (RN absent)	34.8	105.1	(3.03)
3 workers (RN absent)	37.2	110.8	(2.98)
1 worker (RN present)	33.4	93.1	(2.78)
2 workers (RN present)	35.0	108.5	(3.10)
3 workers (RN present)	36.7	131.1	(3.57)
Two-Man Partnership			
2 workers (RN absent)	33.3	91.0	(2.73)
3 workers (RN absent)	36.3	113.4	(3.12)
2 workers (RN present)	34.7	112.7	(3.25)
3 workers (RN present)	36.4	116.6	(3.20)
4 workers (RN present)	36.5	123.9	(3.39)
5 workers (RN present)	38.7	127.9	(3.31)
Three-Man Group			
4 workers (RN present)	35.2	108.6	(3.09)
5+ workers (RN present)	38.4	126.1	(3.28)
Four-Man Group			
5+ workers (RN present)	38.5	115.9	(3.01)
Five or More (Multispecialty) Group			
5+ workers (RN present)	37.3	105.1	(2.82)

Source: Yankauer et al. (1970b), p. 39. Data is for October 1967.

One piece of evidence regarding productivity by hospital staff physicians is available from data published in *Hospital Physician.* (See Table 7-9.) This data indicates that, with the exception of general practitioners, productivity is much lower in salaried hospital practice than in the modes outlined above. Although one might expect case mix differences to explain some of the productivity variations,[21] the size of the gaps are still quite large.

Yett (1967) used Medical Economics data from a 1965 survey to investigate economies of scale by means of cost function estimation. His sample consisted of 1262 self-employed physicians under age 65. Defining output, q, as total patient visits per year and costs, C, as tax-deductible professional expenses, he estimated a linear cost function of the form.

$$C = \lambda q. \tag{7.11}$$

Table 7-8
Practice Size and Productivity Relationships

			Visits Per MD Hour			
	4					3.01 (1.25)
Number of MDs					3.09 (1.33)	3.28 (1.66)
in practice **3**						
2		3.25 (1)	3.20 (1.5)	3.39 (2)	3.31 (2.5)	
1	2.78 (1)	3.10 (2)	3.57 (3)			
	1	2	3	4	5+	
			Number of Ancillaries			

Source: Berki (1972), p. 12.

Table 7-9
Hospital Staff Physicians

Field	Direct Hours Worked[a]	Total Hours Worked[b]	Visits[c] Series 1	Visits[c] Series 2
General Practice	33	49	135(4.09)	155(4.70)
General Surgery	33	59	69(2.08)	86(2.61)
Internal Medicine	26	53	52(2.00)	69(2.65)
Pediatricians	21	53	30(1.43)	47(2.24)
All Fields	–	50	–	–

[a]Number of hours full-time hospital staff physicians spent treating patients in the hospital per week during 1966.

[b]Number of hours spent in all professional activity per week during 1966, including private practice.

[c]Series 1 is the median number of visits with the physician's own patients in the hospital. Series 2 includes other physicians' patients treated by the physician in addition to his own in the hospital. Numbers in parentheses are visits per direct hours worked.

Source: *Hospital Physician*, July 1967, pp. 35-39.

This indicated increasing returns to scale over a broad range of output. However, an alternative rate-volume cost function specification

$$C = T_1 q + T_2 \gamma \tag{7.12}$$

yielded much lower estimates of economies of scale over a more narrow output range. The latter implied a much smaller optimum-sized practice. Other results were that expense functions varied by region (East, Midwest, South, and West in ascending order of average expense per patient visit per year) and by broad medical specialty (general practice, medical specialties, and surgical specialties in ascending order as expected).

Taylor and Newhouse (1970) and Newhouse (1973) report overhead costs per patient visit (all nonphysician costs except costs of ancillary services and space) to be far greater in three outpatient clinics ($14.24) than in a small sample of private practice physicians they surveyed ($4.54). Both solo and group practices are included in the private practice sample; the largest of these is considerably smaller (measured in terms of the number of patient visits) than the smallest of the three outpatient clinics. Sloan (1973a, p. 21) reports the average labor cost per visit (including the physician) at three community mental health center outpatient clinics to be $21.93, $52.13, and $27.16 for late 1969 and early 1970. By comparison, the mean charges on a national basis for first and follow-up office visits according to the American Medical Association were $32.64 and $29.50, respectively. The national mean charges presumably cover physician time, other labor, as well as capital costs. Moreover, they refer to individual patient contacts with a psychiatrist. By contrast, most therapist contacts in the three clinics were to groups of patients; each patient contact counted as a visit. Unlike private practice, the therapist in the clinic was often a nonpsychiatrist. Both studies report a substantial amount of time spent by staff in nonpatient related functions. This data suggests a lack of incentive for efficient production within institutional (salaried) practice.

Table 7-10 gives data on practice expenses (excluding the physician) per visit for 1969-1970. These are even lower than the Taylor-Newhouse private practice estimates, in part reflecting definitional differences and because Taylor-New-house's data pertain to a major metropolitan area rather than to the nation as a whole. According to Table 7-10, groups, primarily fee-for-service, have the lowest expense-visit ratio. This data suggests that something other than size *per*

Table 7-10
Weeks Worked, Visits, and Expenses for Visits

Type of Practice	Weeks Worked	Direct Hrs. Worked	Total Hrs. Worked	Visits	Expenses/ Visit
	Physicians in All Fields				
Solo	48.1	45.6	50.9	126.5(2.77)	$3.75
Two-man partnership	48.2	47.9	53.9	158.2(3.30)	3.56
Informal association	48.3	49.1	55.1	132.2(2.69)	3.71
Group	47.8	47.0	53.5	156.4(3.33)	2.97

Notes: Numbers in parentheses in the visits column are the number of visits per hour of patient care (direct hours worked). Weeks worked and expenses correspond to 1969. Hours and visits are for 1970.

Source: Center for Health Services Research and Development (1972).

se may explain the differences between outpatient clinic and private practice expenses. Of course, the comparisons would be somewhat more definitive if the group category were disaggregated by size of practice.

Alternative Reimbursement Schemes

Empirical evidence on the effect of various reimbursement mechanisms on physician productivity is practically nonexistent. (It should be noted that reimbursement here refers to the way in which the physician is compensated for his services, and not the mode used by the patient to pay for services received.) Some tentative findings regarding the impact of expense or cost sharing within group practices were mentioned in the previous section. Sloan (in Chapter 3) has formally developed and posed several hypotheses dealing with the question of incentives within groups. Rigorous tests, unfortunately, were not possible with existing data. Therefore, most of the following section is based upon theoretical considerations. The only possible exception to this lack of empirical work is an extensive cross-country comparison done by Glazer (1970). This work, however, does not include any systematic statistical analyses.

In general, alternative methods of physician reimbursement are expected to provide different incentives for physician behavior. These may affect both the demand for medical services (to the extent that the physician's advice to his patients differs under different reimbursement schemes) and the supply of medical services in terms of physician hours worked.

The three broad methods of reimbursement most frequently discussed are (1) fee-for-service, a piecework basis, (2) salary fixed for some time period, and (3) capitation, an amount per person "assigned" or "treated," fixed for some time period (Pauly, 1970, p. 117). There are many possible combinations of these methods with the various types of practice modes, solo, group, partnership, or staff employment. Regardless of which scheme is used, its effectiveness will generally depend upon three factors: (1) the strength of professional ethics, (2) the range of alternative treatments associated with particular diagnoses, and (3) institutional arrangements. Associated incentives and disincentives will be outlined for each of the above plans.

Under fee-for-service, the physician is paid for each unit of service performed and has the obvious financial incentive to increase both the output of services per unit of input and the total number of services provided. This may take the form of either offering services which are only marginally called for, or, when faced with a choice from a set of potential treatments, selecting the one with the highest marginal revenue (which need not be the least cost procedure) (Monsma, 1970). This incentive to provide extra services is exacerbated in situations where the patient is not responsible for his bill, since the cost to him of the extra service may be low or zero.

Also crucial in a fee-for-service system is the manner in which fees or charges are determined. If prices are fixed by procedure or specialty, then the system risks the dangers inherent in any nonflexible pricing scheme; overutilization of those procedures priced high relative to marginal cost, and underutilization of underpriced services. In the long run, this could lead to a misallocation of the physician stock over various specialties. On the other hand, a flexible pricing system, such as the customary and usual fee method, depends crucially on the physicians' professional ethics, since there are no disincentives to passing on increased costs due to production inefficiency or the adoption of sophisticated (though not necessarily efficacious or cost reducing) technologies. It would seem that formalized peer review mechanisms would have their potentially greatest payoff under this last type of reimbursement arrangement.

Under capitation, the physician is reimbursed in proportion to the number of patients he has agreed to treat over some period of time (usually a year).[22] There is clearly no incentive to provide unnecessary treatments, since payments are not tied to the number of services rendered. Rather, there are incentives both not to provide services, and to provide services at lower costs (and possibly lower quality). It is also likely that because physicians value leisure, they will prefer less laborious and time consuming tasks whenever possible (Pauly, 1970, p. 117). This has the implication that, under capitation, they have a stake to keep their assignees as healthy as possible by employing preventive measures, and to treat cases as early as possible when the costs of treatment are usually lower. The strength of this effect has never been clearly demonstrated, however.

The second factor associated with capitation is the manner in which subscribers are enrolled. Unlike fee-for-service, physicians' incomes are now functions of the number of their subscribers, not the number of services provided. Presumably, competition between physicians will mitigate incentives to either underprovide services or offer poor quality care. However, patients' difficulties in evaluating the quantity and quality of care received, and professional impediments to the dissemination of information make the effectiveness of a competitive control mechanism suspect (Hadley, 1972). Where physicians are organized in groups, competition will depend crucially on the ability of the market to sustain more than one provider.

Salaried reimbursement occupies a middle ground between capitation and fee-for-service. There are no clear incentives to either overprovide or underprovide services. One would suspect, however, that if salary were determined independently of performance, then only the minimum quantity and quality of services necessary to retain one's position would be offered. On the other hand, if next period's salary depended on the number of procedures performed in the current period, then the incentive effects would be similar to those of fee-for-service (Pauly, 1970, p. 118). On a national level, one should also be concerned with the salary *structure*, both within the medical profession and relative to other professions. In the long run, there would likely be effects on the quality, quantity, and distribution of new physicians.

Attempting to assess the productivity implications of each of these schemes is beset with measurement problems, value judgments, and the ambiguous movements of inputs and quality. Presumably, fee-for-service induces increases in all three of input, output, and quality, capitation results in decreases, and salaries have no clear implications. In comparing fee-for-service and capitation, the issues of which overtreats and which undertreats can only be discussed in the context of society's (or the individual's) *valuation* of extra units of medical care. Sloan has collected some data relating major sources of income to hours supplied and productivity (see Table 7-11), but this data should be considered only suggestive, since it allows no way of accounting for differences in physician tastes for types of practices, for adverse prior selection, or for variations in case mix. One would suspect, however, because of the very large differences in productivity between salaried and fee-for-service reimbursement, that there are some incentive effects being picked up.

Sloan has also asked the more specific question of the effects of cost-sharing and income-cost-sharing within group practices upon output, prices, and input purchase decisions. Based upon careful theoretical development, he formulates a number of hypotheses.

... Cost-sharing physicians should set quantity higher and price lower than their non-cost-sharing colleagues. However, the incentive to reduce costs is lower under cost-sharing and this incentive diminishes as the size of the group increases. If the cost parameters vary directly with group size, which is plausible, quantity is lower and price higher. Income-(revenue-cost) sharing groups may take several forms. Apportioning net practice income for the group among physicians equally, the model predicts that output will be lower for higher group size; it will also be lower if costs imputed by the physician are higher. Price varies directly with both group size and the imputed costs. As in cost-sharing practices, the income gain to the individual physicians from a reduction in either

Table 7-11
Hours Worked and Visits per Week

Major Source of Income	Patient Care Hours Worked	Total Hours Worked	Visits
Fee-for-service only	47.1	52.3	141.8(3.0)
Fee-for-service with some salary	43.7	51.4	123.0(2.8)
Salary with some fee-for-service	35.3	48.3	98.1(2.8)
Salary only	34.9	46.6	102.7(2.9)
Retainer only	43.0	44.0	102.8(2.4)

Note: Numbers in parentheses in the visits column are the number of visits per hour of patient care. Hours and visits are for 1970.
Source: Center for Health Services Research and Development (1972).

fixed and/or marginal costs is negative. Unequal demand for individual members within the equal sharing group does not alter these conclusions. But, equal sharing will not be attractive to the physician with high relative demand and/or low costs.

Numerous types of unequal income-sharing schemes exist. Individual members may receive unequal shares of the total net income of the group, or greater weight (than $1/n$) may be given to revenues and cost attributed to each individual member with a correspondingly lower weight on the net income generated by other group members.[23] The former method mitigates the disincentive effects of large group size for members receiving more than $1/n$ of group net revenue, but increases it for those who receive a smaller proportion than $1/n$. Weighting the individual contribution more heavily raises quantity, lowers price, and raises physician cost-consciousness. However, it also increases the variance in individual member income which would not be desirable to the risk averse physician.

Using Section II-type models, salaried practice appears very unattractive. Effort should fall to a minimum "acceptable" level. Moreover, there is no incentive under this arrangement for individual physicians to monitor costs. Prepayment retainer practices are distinguished by having a group demand schedule rather than a set of schedules for individual members. These ways of specifying demand are not fully appropriate for either practice arrangement, but there is a tendency for demand under prepayment to be more oriented toward the group than under fee-for-service practice. The major consequence of group demand is that individual member output depends (negatively) on the output of other members. This factor would tend to equalize effort among members. However, disincentive effects associated with size remain (Sloan, 1973a, pp. 11-12).

Unfortunately, existing data does not permit rigorous testing of these hypotheses. About the most that Sloan can say is that disincentive and decreasing cost-consciousness effects need not occur if group members find a method for representing their collective interests. Looking at the proportion of groups which employ a manager or board of directors indicates that this is in fact what occurs. As group size increases, the proportion with managers also increases, becoming greater than fifty percent at a size of five members (Sloan, 1973a, p. 14). The proportion is also generally higher for multispecialty groups, where effective peer monitoring may be difficult, than for single specialty or general practice groups. Looking at methods for distributing income, fixed salaries was a quantitatively insignificant reimbursement scheme, including generally less than 4 percent of the groups considered (p. 16). Finally, multispecialty groups were much more likely to have unequal share plans than single specialty or general practice groups. The likelihood of unequal shares also increases with group size for multispecialty groups.

Effects of Licensure on
Manpower Productivity

Economists interested in examining the effects of licensure upon the medical care system have tended to direct their research at one of two questions: (1) the effect of variations in licensure barriers on physician and dentist mobility, and (2) the costs of licensure resulting from physicians' purported monopolistic behavior.[24] The former work has concluded that mobility barriers are practically nonexistent for physicians, and perhaps somewhat stronger for dentists, while the latter has been inconclusive. Although each of the above has indirect implications for manpower productivity, the effects of licensure have not been directly investigated. Therefore, this section, based largely on the chapter by Ted Frech, will present a theoretical summary of the areas in which licensure may effect productivity. Since the power to license health personnel is located primarily at the state level of government, it may be convenient to begin by looking at licensure productivity implications within any particular jurisdiction. We shall then examine the possible effects of interstate variations in licensure conditions.

It might also be helpful to note at this time that although the terms accreditation, licensure, and certification are closely related and often used interchangeably, they do have different meanings and should be distinguished from each other. Accreditation refers to the process by which an agency or organization evaluates and recognizes an institution or program of study as meeting certain predetermined criteria or standards. Licensure involves the process by which an agency or government grants permission to persons to practice in a given profession by attesting that those licensed have attained the minimal degree of competency necessary to ensure that the public health, safety, and welfare will be reasonably protected. Certification deals with the process by which a nongovernmental agency or association grants recognition to an individual who has met certain predetermined qualifications specified by that agency or association (Dean, 1972, p. 6).

Because of the tremendous growth in the numbers and types of health personnel over the last two decades, states have had varying degrees of difficulty in keeping their licensing laws up-to-date with new health manpower categories, and in clearly distinguishing between their functions and job specifications. This rapid growth can be illustrated by the fact that in 1930 only seven programs of study in the health field were accredited: medicine, osteopathy, dentistry, podiatry, nursing, occupational therapy, and physical therapy; by 1970, the number exceeded thirty. Another striking illustration of the growth in training activities is the fact that while in 1950 there were approximately 140,000 allied health workers in the country, by 1970 that number had soared to 535,000 (Dean, 1972, p. 8). While in most cases the laws are fairly clear on who is to be licensed, they are frequently very vague regarding precisely what these persons can do.

Another problem is created by the fact that licensing statutes are often very rigid in their educational and experience requirements, and usually do not permit credit for on-the-job training or other methods of acquiring requisite performance skills and knowledge. Some of this rigidity, however, is slowly being relaxed. For example, California now recognizes equivalency qualifications for medical corpsmen who want to become registered nurses, applicants seeking licensure as vocational nurses, and licensed vocational nurses who want to become registered nurses. In New York, the law provides that experience and training other than that traditionally prescribed may be used as alternative qualifications for examination in X-ray technology (Dean, 1972, p. 16).

Finally, most state laws make no provision for assuring the maintenance of competency by licensees. Obtaining a license is basically a one-shot affair, and once granted one is virtually assured of lifetime authorization to practice his profession, regardless of whether he/she maintains performance capabilities or keeps abreast of advancements in his/her field (Dean, 1972, p. 17).

What are the implications for manpower productivity? It was noted earlier that there appear to be substantial potential productivity gains in the increased utilization of ancillary personnel. It seems fairly obvious that one possible reason why these economies have not been fully realized may lie in restrictive licensure laws. In effect, restrictions on which types of personnel may perform what tasks prevent the technically (and economically) efficient solution from being attained. These laws prevent the substitution of generally less intensively trained manpower for more expensive manpower inputs, especially physicians and dentists. Inefficiencies of this sort are likely to arise not only in physicians' offices, but also in clinics, hospitals, and group practices. Further, where delegation to lower level personnel is permitted, the laws may be overly restrictive regarding supervisory restrictions and ultimate legal responsibility.

The lack of proficiency and equivalency procedures is likely to have two effects, one operating through upward career mobility, and the other affecting the nature of prospective entrants to the health professions. Blocking upward ladders to higher paying and higher status professions is likely to have disincentives for self-improvement and continuing education by lower level personnel. For most people, returning to school to meet formal requirements would not be economically rational.[25] Further, those who do acquire additional competence would tend to have their skills underutilized. In addition, the inability to move upwards has the effect of lowering expected lifetime income at each entry point into the health professions. On the basis of the theory of human capital and its implications for occupational choice, and given the generally acknowledged correlation between innate ability and expected incomes, one would expect, on average, a lower qualified individual to select a particular health profession that has limited upward mobility.

Finally, the lack of retesting or periodic competency reviews would also appear to reduce incentives for continuing education. The impact of this may be greatest for physicians, who are faced with a continually and rapidly expanding body of new knowledge and new techniques. The implication, then, is that the quality of care provided would be higher than under existing procedures. On the other side of the coin, current statutes make it exceedingly difficult to weed out obviously incompetent practitioners.

The effects on productivity of interstate variations in licensure seem to be twofold. Although most empirical work by economists has shown licensure barriers to have a negligible impact on physician mobility, this is not the case for other levels of health manpower, from dentists on down. However, barriers are perhaps strongest for physicians who are graduates of foreign medical schools, and who currently comprise a large fraction of our physician manpower. To some extent, therefore, licensure barriers would seem to be the source of artificial surpluses and shortages of health manpower, and their consequent inefficient utilization.

The second problem has to do with the wide variation in the number of health occupations which are licensed in various states, and with variations in the legal job descriptions for particular job titles. In addition to hindering mobility, these differences lead to considerable confusion as to who has authority to do what. Secondly, many new types of health professions (e.g., physician assistants, MEDEX, nurse practitioners) are being developed. It is highly conceivable that people will be trained in these areas, only to face limited job markets due to the failure of many states to pass the requisite amendments to their licensure laws.

Changes in the Quality and Distribution
of Medical Manpower

It has been known for some time that there are variations in physician productivity across specialties, geographic areas, and community sizes. For example, from *Medical Economics'* quadrennial surveys of physicians, we observe, for the year 1970, rates of patient visits per week of approximately 175 for general practice, 120 for internal medicine, 155 internal medicine, 155 for pediatrics, 110 for general surgery, and 130 for obstetrics-gynecology. On a regional basis the rates are 118, 158, 156, and 120 for the east, south, midwest, and west, respectively. Table 7-12 further illustrates some of the variations in productivity.

To some extent, of course, these figures reflect differences inherent in the medical nature of the specialties. The average surgical procedure is likely to require more time than, say, the average gynecological examination. There may also be some differences in the average degree of necessity or difficulty associated with cases treated by various specialists. For example, pediatricians are generally acknowledged to perform a good deal of well-child care. Productivity rates across geographic areas are likely to depend upon physician specialty composition and case-mix differences. Thus, we would expect the more esoteric types of specialists and more severe types of cases to be located in urban rather than rural areas. Finally, people's attitudes and values toward medical care and broad physician attitudes toward treatment modalities may differ across the country, and may have some effect upon measured productivity rates.

Table 7-12
Variations in Patient-Visit Rates by Location (Patient Visits per Private Physicians per Week)

	Urban	Suburban	Rural	All
East	112	121	–	118
South	137	161	250	158
Midwest	144	150	179	156
West	110	128	–	120
National	124	137	181	137

Ranges of Total Patient Visits in Five Major Fields

	GPs	Internists	General Surgeons	OBGs	Pediatricians
250 or more	23%	7%	5%	6%	13%
175-249	29	14	13	18	26
150-174	17	12	12	14	16
125-149	9	16	17	17	16
100-124	6	16	19	21	13
75-99	6	18	15	13	9
50-74	4	11	12	8	6
Fewer than 50	3	6	7	3	1

Source: *Medical Economics* (January 18, 1971), pp. 87, 89. Copyright © 1971 by Medical Economics Company, Oradell, N.J. 07649. Reprinted by permission.

However, there is a growing body of somewhat fragmentary evidence that these rate differences may be the result of varying incentives for physicians to be efficient in the delivery of medical care. Roemer (1961, p. 991) found a strong inverse correlation between the physician-population ratio of a state and an adjusted (for insurance coverage and bed supply) hospital admission rate. He argued that this was caused by differences in the relative supplies and demands for physician services across states. As demands on a physician's time increase, he has to devise methods to deal with more patients per unit of time. One such method is to hospitalize patients who, under other demand conditions, could be treated on an ambulatory basis. In the hospital, the physician is partially subsidized by the hospital's staff and resources, and he/she can generally see several patients in the time required to see one in the office. [While this may be efficient from the individual physician's point of view, it is probably more costly from society's perspective because of the higher costs of hospitalization (Feldstein, 1971, pp. 864-65).] Rafferty (1971) found a similar result for the way in which hospitals respond to fluctuations in the demand for hospital beds. As the hospital occupancy rate goes up, average case-specific lengths of stay go up as well, implying that more severe or necessary types of cases are being given priority over postponable cases. (In terms of the above discussion dealing with output measurement, this would mean that "real" output, as opposed to measured output, e.g., cases or admissions, has gone up. If inputs were held constant, then real productivity would also increase.)

The implicit hypothesis in each of these works is that pressures or incentives for physicians to be efficient are a positive function of the degree of *excess* demand in particular areas and/or specialties. (Note that excess demand refers to the *difference* between the quantities demanded and supplied, not the absolute level of demand.) This hypothesis is also supported by the casual observations that regional productivity rates are inversely correlated with regional physician-population ratios, which may be considered a crude measure of relative supply and demand, and by the findings by Riddick et al. (1971) and Yankauer et al. (1970b) that utilization of ancillary personnel, which is presumably productivity increasing, is also inversely correlated with regional differences in excess demand.

These observations suggest that one way to increase physician productivity would be through a reallocation of physicians from low productivity specialties, geographic areas and/or community sizes to high productivity areas. If the medical care production function is subject to decreasing marginal and average productivity (as seems intuitively the case) then such redistribution would be consistent with a reallocation from activities in *relative* surplus to activities in *relative* shortage. While it is true that some areas, etc., might suffer a net reduction, or at least a reduced rate of increase in physician availability, the higher productivity in the areas to which physicians would be reallocated would more than offset those losses. (In more technical terms, this is simply an application of the general efficiency criterion that additional units of input be allocated such that marginal products per dollar, adjusted for inherent differences, be equal across all activities.) Such a reallocation should also have the effect of increasing equity in the availability of physician services.

Reallocation could come about by either altering the existing distribution of the *stock* of physicians and/or the *flow* of new physicians from medical schools. The theory of human capital, however, suggests that physicians with established practices would have relatively high "move" prices. In fact, rough calculations by Sloan indicate that the costs of altering the stock distribution would be so high as to be politically unfeasible (Sloan, 1968). Further, there have been one or two studies of physicians who have actually changed their specialty and/or location (Crawford and McCormack, 1971; Mathis, 1969). It appears, unfortunately, that those most ripe for moves prefer to move in the "wrong" direction, i.e., towards greater specialization and more urban locations. Therefore, reallocation attempts would seem to be best directed at new physicians.

Once focus has been trained on new physicians, a second general tack comes to mind. Policy may also be directed at raising the quality (i.e., the *marginal* productivity) of new entrants to the health professions. Further, there are several dimensions along which policy intervention could occur: application to medical school, admissions criteria, medical school curricula, the length of medical education, and the nature and form of postgraduate training. For example, medical schools could develop courses in practice management and patient relationships which make graduates more practice oriented and more efficiency conscious. However, much is still unknown about many of the relevant structural relationships. How are specialty and location choices related to individuals' backgrounds, to their medical school curricula, to the general school environment, and to external economic incentives? While not still fully resolved, work on location choice indicates that the probability of a new physician locating in a particular state is a positive function of the number and proximity of previous contacts with that state (Yett and Sloan, 1972). From a broader perspective, physician migratory behavior seems to be fairly coincident with the migration pattern of the white male population in general (Held, 1972), which has tended to follow what we might call "economic pull" incentives. The direction of causation, however, between economic incentives and population flows is not fully clear. For an occupational group as small as physicians, though, this problem is probably not analytically important.

The relationship between quality and medical education is probably far more complex, and far less is known about it. A major part of the problem stems from our inability to precisely define physician quality. Intuitively, both innate ability and the quality of medical education should have a positive effect on physician performance. However, attempts to verify such a relationship empirically have not yet had any great success (Peterson et al., 1963). Here again much more can be said about areas for research than about behavioral and structural relationships upon which policy recommendation can be based.

Technical Change

The study of the role played by technical change in increasing manpower productivity has had a long history in economics, but is very new to the area of medical economics. With the exception of Weisbrod's 1971 study of the costs and benefits generated by polio research, there has been little work on either the process by which new medical knowledge and technologies are generated, or the ways they diffuse into general use. Nor have there been any rigorous attempts to relate technical change to manpower productivity. Therefore, this section is limited to a number of general comments which attempt to highlight some relevant aspects of medical technical change. These lead to suggestions for future research.

It has generally been assumed that advances in technology unambiguously increases productivity. However, there may be at least two reasons why this assumption might not always hold for medical care. The first stems from the fact that health and disease are basically adaptive concepts, changing to suit the external environment (Boulding, 1966). Thus as knowledge expands and better medical techniques are developed, it is likely that the *average* complexity and/or severity of medical cases will go up over time. It is also likely that a good deal of technology is engaging in a tradeoff between mortality and morbidity. In Thomas' terms, there has been a shift from curative and preventive to maintenance technology (1971). In general we would expect this shift in case-mix to result in a more resource-intensive type of case. Therefore, many of our productivity measures are likely to decline, rather than increase, as a consequence of technical changes. Of course, in large part, this reflects our inability to measure changes in health status, which presumably has gone up. However, to the extent that we don't know the relative valuation of mortality and morbidity, even that may be somewhat unclear.

The second difficulty with the usual assumption about the relationship between technical change and productivity stems from the peculiar environment provided by the medical care market; most innovators and adopters of new technology are not subject to market profitability tests. In a regime of full cost reimbursement there is little incentive to develop or adopt resource-saving types of technology. Rather, the emphasis appears to have been on sophisticated, quality increasing types of innovations, which also, unfortunately, tend to increase resource requirements. Because of the lack of market competition, there has been no real necessity to demonstrate either the increased efficiency or efficacy of new systems as compared to what they were replacing. For example, there has been some recent evidence indicating that intensive care procedures for heart attack victims may have only a marginal impact on survival rates, compared to the previous technology for treating heart patients.[26]

All this suggests that there may be room for public intervention into the process by which new products and processes are developed and adopted. However, it is not at all clear what kind of mechanism, if any, would provide effective controls or incentives. The conflict between "directed" and "nondirected" research programs, and the experience of the cancer and sickle cell anemia programs, illustrate the inadequacy of our knowledge.

Suggested Research

What we would like to know often appears limitless. But the increasingly important role of research and experimentation in policy formation, in the legislative process, and in actual government management, makes it essential that efforts be expended to identify and discuss the more promising avenues for future work.

Ancillary Personnel

Many of the observations about potential productivity gains were based upon estimated production functions. It was clear, however, that the results were sensitive to the type of function chosen. Therefore, more work needs to be done on specifying and estimating physician production functions, and it is important that this work be extended to finer classifications of medical specialties and modes of organization. This suggests that, rather than more macroproduction function studies, we need a series of microeconomic studies of the physician production process. Input-output analysis may be very useful in this context.

We also need more work on the range of tasks which technically *could* be delegated to ancillaries, as well as observations on actual delegation patterns. Where there are divergences, and it is likely that these may be considerable, possible causes should be investigated. As part of this same general topic, delegation patterns across the various institutional settings of medical care delivery should be examined. Do allied health personnel perform the same tasks in hospitals, ambulatory clinics, and large group practices as in physicians' offices? If not, does one type of setting appear to employ them more efficiently.

Barriers to greater utilization of ancillaries should be explored. Of primary importance in this area is the relationship between licensure and utilization. Also of interest is the effect of excess demand for physicians' services upon incentives to expand task delegation and ancillary employment.

We should also know a good deal more about the labor market for allied health professionals. What kinds of people are drawn into these occupations? Are occupational choices sensitive to fluctuations in net rates of return? Do rates of return accurately reflect relative surpluses and shortages for ancillaries over geographic areas and various types of institutions? Finally, can profit-making training institutions be called upon to respond to the needs for new types of ancillaries, or is initial federal subsidization of training called for?

Capital Substitution

The capital substitution literature reviewed above appeared to be deficient in at least three ways. First, insufficient attention was paid to the question of economic feasibility. Future experiments involving capital-based systems should be required to evaluate the annual operating cost of the equipment, including depreciation and the cost of support personnel, savings realized by reduced requirements of other inputs, and both the quantity and value of the increased output, if any. Assessing output value and determining the impact on quality of care appear to be related tasks. Quality parameters, such as the change in blood sugar used by Reiffen and Komaroff (1972), should be developed. Or one could attempt to relate the increased output to the length of inpatient stays, the number of disability days, visit intervals, or mortality rates. Under these conditions one might hope to make successful comparisons of a system's effectiveness, at least relative to the prior mode.

The second shortcoming of the literature reviewed is its inattention to incentives for adopting new capital equipment. If capital substitution does in fact raise productivity and lower costs, are there any assurances that such capital would be accepted by the relevant institutions? Are there particular characteristics of institutions, physicians, and/or administrators which distinguish adopters from nonadopters? How does the external incentive structure affect an institution's capital purchasing decisions? For example, one could compare how hospital capital intensity and mix vary under full cost reimbursement, cost plus reimbursement, profit maximization (proprietary hospitals), and public control (short-term VA hospitals). Such a study, of course, would have to control or attempt to hold case mix constant. It would be of special interest to determine how demand pressures, as measured by, say, occupancy or patient visit rates, affect the capital decisions of hospitals, clinics, group practices, and other private practitioners.

Finally, not enough research has been done on the productivity-increasing potential of noncomputer based capital. All of the above questions should also be asked of both the esoteric and more mundane types of capital. In particular, it would be interesting to compare the diffusion patterns of capital which originates in the private, profit-making medical equipment industry with capital developed through public and other nonprofit R&D. Is medical capital sold through the same kinds of intensive marketing techniques commonly associated with drug sales? Are there the same problems of nonefficacious equipment? Given the tremendous growth in the value of capital equipment and its seemingly high potential for achieving cost reductions, all of these questions are of increasing importance.

Increased Patient Involvement

As indicated by Golladay in Chapter 4, three major research thrusts are required if the economic implications of patient participation in health care are to be assessed systematically. First, the areas of desirable behavioral change must be identified. Second, the determinants of behavior must be ascertained. And third, effective programs for affecting behavioral change through the determinants of behavior must be develped and evaluated. There appears a priori to be considerable independence among health problems with respect to each of these issues, which suggests that each major category of health problem might be considered independently of other problems.

The first thrust proposed here would seek to identify potentially cost-effective modes of patient participation. These modes are of three types: (1) health maintenance, (2) compliance, and (3) self-care. The notion of health maintenance although intuitively appealing has not been subjected to serious economic analysis. It would be useful to evaluate the optimal level of health maintenance as opposed to episodic care, and the sensitivity of solution values to the prices of medical services and the opportunity cost of patient supplied inputs. Such an investigation would compare the cost-effectiveness of preventive care and early diagnosis with that of treatment of symptomic conditions. It is not obvious, given the costs of prevention or screening, that preventive modes are superior to episodic modes of care. Resolution of this issue would indicate areas in which patient education is potentially productive and would provide insights into the role of health maintenance activities in reducing the cost of medical care. An incidental outcome would be an indication of the optimal periodicity for screening and asymptomic diagnosis. The proposed analysis obviously must distinguish patient strata wherever risk factors can be identified.

The second research effort would focus on the problem of noncompliance. The existing literature documents the extent of noncompliance but fails to either indicate the consequences of the misbehavior or to identify its correlates. It would be useful to know whether noncompliance is a genuine problem in the management of conditions or merely an affront to the provider. Furthermore, if patient education is to be evaluated as an instrument for effecting greater compliance, it is necessary to determine the reasons for noncompliance. The literature suggest that ignorance and misinformation are major sources of the problem but provides little systematic defense for the view. Two sets of studies are proposed, therefore. The first would extend the investigations of compliance studies to evaluate the impact of specific types of noncompliance on the effectiveness of professional care. The second would examine the determinants as opposed to the correlates of noncompliance; in particular, it would seek to go behind socioeconomic identifiers in an attempt to isolate attitudes or beliefs which produce noncompliant behavior.

The third research effort would investigate cost-effective methods of patient education in both hospital and outpatient settings. As indicated above, the existing literature on the pedagogy of health education is largely anecdotal. A cost-effectiveness type of evaluative research would therefore be useful, in order to determine whether education is a viable method for confronting health problems. This research should recognize the differences in learning abilities, language usage, and intellectual backgrounds of strata of patients in order to tailor educational experiences to individuals and hence to increase learning effectiveness. It is likely that much of the proposed analysis could rely upon existing operational programs of health education and participation for data.

Finally, a professional reassessment of the role of the patient in self-care would be useful. It seems likely that a careful review of opportunities for delegation of tasks to patients or patients' households would be suggestive of new modes of care. This exercise seems particularly appropriate in the face of widespread interest in the introduction of new paraprofessions into the health care team. The notion that persons with limited formal training should be delegated some responsibilities previously reserved by the physician, also suggests that patients might be delegated some of these functions.

The opportunities for cost-effective participation of patients in the provision of health care are most likely to appear in chronic, long-term conditions, or frequently recurring problems. The foregoing research issues should be considered first for such chronic problems as diabetes, cardiovascular disease, and kidney failure; second priority should be attached to common, recurrent problems such as upper respiratory infections and minor trauma.

Group Practice, Other Practice Modes, and Alternative Reimbursement Schemes

Much remains to be learned about the structure of incentives in medical practice, how they vary according to group size, and what the effects of alternative incentives on medical practice performance are. If output, price, and input cost decisions are made by individual members, one should expect a loss in efficiency. Fortunately, group decision-making seems to become more important as the number of physician members increases. However, more detailed data are needed to verify current impressions. Our knowledge of the effect of incentives will remain quite limited until more specific information is gathered on internal incentives in various types of practices as well as on factors leading to physician choices of specific practice modes. If group practice managers and boards of directors do in fact impose cost consciousness upon group members, then their behavior should also be studied, particularly the relative effects of salary and profit sharing reimbursement for managers.

There are several other interesting and important questions involving incentives. First, there is a need for research describing how decisions with respect to input purchases, physician effort, and pricing are made in various practice settings. Much of this information can be obtained from direct questions. Researchers have preferred to infer inefficiencies indirectly from empirical cost functions, but the indirect approach gives only general indications of inefficiency, at best, and it does not allow one to locate its source. Second, studies of practice mode choices would be useful. To date, there has been no effort to gather information on preferences for groups of specific sizes. Moreover, available data focuses on practice preferences, but there has been no emphasis on studying characteristics of physicians who made specific practice mode decisions in the recent past. The latter type of analysis may be more fruitful because it is difficult to capture the intensity of practice preferences. The third type of study concerns the effect of the incentives on performance. It would be useful to measure intervening variables as well as output, prices, and input costs under alternative incentive structures. For example, what type of information is gathered in alternative practice settings before a major capital purchase is made? Specifically, how does the physician's work schedule change as n increases? In sum, emphasis in future research on this and related issues should be much more detailed than it has been to date.

Licensure

Almost all the observations made in the section on licensure were based on either theoretical or intuitive ground. Therefore, many of those points should have empirical verification. In particular, a comparative analysis of manpower behavior with respect to task assignment and delegation under various degrees of licensure conditions might give us a better idea of the extent to which licensure regulations actually create barriers to efficient manpower utilization. The literature suggested that there were considerable interstate variations in the numbers of health professions licensed, the restrictiveness of licensing conditions, and the definitions of health occupations. One might investigate the relationships between these factors and ancillary utilization and task delegation.

Implicit in much of the discussion underlying licensure and credentialing is the assumption that there is a positive relationship between formal education or training and manpower performance. This certainly lies behind arguments supporting continuing education for physicians. However, the real value of such programs has not fully been explored, nor have various means of providing continuing education been examined. For example, comparing the performance (by some criteria) of roughly similar physicians who undertake varying amounts of extra education would be interesting. This could be extended to include the worth of board certification. Also, a study of the extent and value of the education provided by group practices would help in assessing both the group practice mode and continuing education.

Changes in Medical Manpower

Here there are three main areas of concern: (1) the specialty-location distribution of physicians, (2) the quality of new manpower entering the health field, and (3) the impact of medical education (and other professional training) on quality and distribution. For a number of reasons, it seems that research should be primarily directed at new entrants. More needs to be known about the relative influences of personal background, medical education, and external economic (and other environmental) factors in medical school graduates' (and other health professionals') specialty-location choices. In particular, policy manipulable variables need to be identified, and the costs of altering the distribution by some given amount should be calculated. Can good predictors of these choices be developed, and can they be used by training and/or health planning institutions to select candidates for medical training?

As in other cases, the quality issue is probably most complex. First, methods for measuring quality and physician performance need to be developed. While we intuitively feel that innate ability has some positive relationship to performance, there is not yet any solid evidence confirming this. Nor do we know very much about how the content of medical education affects quality.

If support of medical education is to become a part of our national health policy, then we should attempt to find out something about the differential effects of various support instruments (student loans and fellowships, block institutional training grants and loans, capitation payments). How are the size and socioeconomic distribution of the applicant pool affected? The rapid increase in federal support of biomedical research appears to have had an impact on medical education; what would be the effect of training grant support?

Finally, many medical schools are now beginning to deviate from the traditional course content of their programs. An analysis of the outcomes (in terms of specialty-location choices and physician performance) would be of great value. This may provide a way of evaluating both the traditional course content of medical education, and the traditional prior preparation of medical students.

Technical Change

We are interested in biomedical R&D and technical change in at least two dimensions, (1) how it directly affects the production function through either process or product innovation, and (2) how it affects the quality of health manpower through expansions in medical knowledge and in what is taught in medical schools and other training institutions. These in turn suggest two basic research questions. First, how do significant advances in medical knowledge and technique come about, and how are they diffused and transmitted to medical care delivery units? Second, how can we evaluate the contribution of technology to productivity? (A careful distinction must be made here between health and medical services as our measures of output.) It is not at all certain that recent technology has really bought us anything except increased costs.

There are several potential research strategies. None of them, unfortunately, are perfect. One is to follow Weisbrod's methodology in his cost benefit analysis of poliomyelitis vaccine. Another is to trace particular diseases over time, noting how treatment has changed, and attempting to relate that to changes in something like disability, mortality rates, etc. Third, several comparison studies could be done of different types of innovations, each perhaps representing a different technological category, such as drugs, capital equipment, and organizational changes.

Notes

1. The major adjustment necessitated by altering the unit of analysis is that factors external to the decision and choice processes at lower levels of analysis become internalized for larger units.

2. The questions of what determines the "right or proper" mix of outputs and the correct distribution are highly complex, and not really appropriate here.

3. DHEW, NIH, Bureau of Health Manpower Education, Division of Manpower Intelligence, unpublished material; Theodore, Sutter, and Haug (1967); and the Distribution of Physicians Series (Chicago: American Medical Association, various years); Health Manpower Source Book; HEW Trends.

4. See Scheffler (1972) for a good brief discussion of some of these issues.

5. The term fractionation is from Klarman (1970), p. 27. It refers to the breaking down of a bundle of medical services formerly considered a single unit into a series of separate services, each with its own charge.

6. Final Report of the Federal Council for Science and Technology, Committee on Automation Opportunities in the Service Areas, Panel on Health Services, Vernon E. Wilson, MD, Chairman (Washington: unpublished report, May 1972), p. 6.

7. See Bernard S. Bloom and Osler L. Peterson, "End Results, Cost and Productivity of Coronary Care Units," *New England Journal of Medicine* (January 11, 1973), 72-78.

8. This estimate was made by Ronald Klar, Office of the Assistant Secretary for Health and Scientific Affairs, DHEW.

9. Some of the other factors affecting relative prices would be shifts in the demands for the products and changes in the production technology.

10. Wilson Report, p. 23.

11. Human Resources Research Center, University of Southern California, "An Original Comparative Analysis of Group Practice and Solo Fee-For-Service Practice," under Contract No. HSM 110-70-354; and Frank A. Sloan, University of Florida, "An Analysis of Physician Price and Output Decisions," under Grant No. HS 00825-01.

12. Given the earlier discussion of quality, it should be clear that productivity would also increase if output quality increased or if required input quality decreased for given quantities of outputs and inputs. However, as was stated then, these possibilities will not be explicitly treated because of the inherent measurement problems involved.

13. As will be seen later, this notion of holding all factors but one constant can be extended to include organizational or technological changes as well as direct alteration of the inputs.

14. Their data was from the AMA's Sixth Periodic Survey of Physicians (1970) and included private practice physicians in various practice arrangements.

15. Memo from Dr. J. Butler, Acting Director, Office of Manpower Development, HRA, February 2, 1973.

16. "The Legal Status of Physician's Assistants," *Hospital Progress*, (October 1972), p. 45.

17. ABT Associates, Inc. is performing a study of the adoption, diffusion, and utilization of several types of major capital equipment in a group of metropolitan hospitals. Results of the study are expected by early 1975. BHSR, Contract No. HSM 110-73-513.

18. Fuchs and Kramer (1972); Gross (1972); Nelson (1972).

19. David Mechanic, "The Sociology of Medicine: Viewpoints and Perspectives," *Journal of Health and Human Behavior*, Vol. 7, No. 4 (1966); and "The Concept of Illness Behavior," *Journal of Chronic Disease*, Vol. 15, No. 2 (1962) 189-94; Barbara Blackwell, "Anticipated Premedical Care Activities of Upper Middle Class Adults and Their Implications for Health Education Practice," *Health Education Monographs*, No. 17 (1962); and see particularly Sam Schulman and Anne M. Smith, "The Concept of Health Among Spanish-Speaking Villagers of New Mexico and Colorado," *Journal of Health and Human Behavior*, Vol. 4, No. 4 (1963); and Derek L. Phillips, "Self-Reliance and Inclination to Adopt the Sick Role," *Social Forces*, Vol. 43, No. 4 (1965) 555-63.

20. For Convenience, M and T will be dropped from the production function notation.

21. Discussion accompanying the data indicates that hospital physicians treat the generally more difficult referral cases.

22. One should keep this system conceptually distinct from prepaid group practice plans, which are generically insurance schemes, not plans for reimbursing physicians. Within a prepaid group practice, physicians could be paid under any combination of a number of different payment methods.

23. n = size of the group.

24. See Sloan (1968); Yett and Sloan (1972); Benham, Maurizi, and Reder (1968); Friedman and Kuznets (1945); and Kessel (1958).

25. This follows from implications of the theory of human capital.

26. B.S. Bloom and O.L. Peterson, "End Results, Cost and Productivity of Coronary-Care Units," *The New England Journal of Medicine* (Jan. 11, 1973), pp. 72-78.

Bibliography

Adamson, T.E., "Critical Issues in the Use of Physician Associates and Assistants," *American Journal of Public Health*, Vol. 61: 1765-79 (September 1971).

Bailey, R.M., "A Comparison of Internists in Solo and Fee-for-Service Group Practice in the San Francisco Bay Area," *Bulletin of the New York Academy of Medicine*, Vol. 44: 1293-1303 (November 1968).

_____ , "Economies of Scale in Medical Practice," in *Empirical Studies in Health Economics*, edited by Herbert E. Klarman. Baltimore: The Johns Hopkins Press, 1970.

Barnett, G.O., "Computers in Patient Care." *New England Journal of Medicine*, Vol. 279: 1321-27 (December 1968).

Benham, L.; A. Maurizi; and M.W. Reder, "Migration, Location, and Remuneration of Medical Personnel: Physicians and Dentists," *Review of Economics and Statistics*, Vol. 50: 332-47 (August 1968).

Bergman, A.B.; S.W. Dassel; and R.J. Wedgwood, "Time-Motion Study of Practicing Pediatricians," *Pediatrics*, Vol. 38: 254-63 (August 1966).

Berkeley Scientific Laboratories, *A Study of Automated Clinical Laboratory Systems.* Rockville, Md.: USDHEW, PHS, HSMHA, DHEW Publication No. (HSM) 72-3004, 1971.

Berki, S.E., "The Economies of New Types of Health Personnel," paper read at the Macy Conference on Intermediate-Level Health Personnel in the Delivery of Direct Health Services. Williamsburg, Virginia (November 12-14, 1972).

Blackwell, Barbara, "The Literature of Delay in Seeking Medical Care for Chronic Illness," *Health Education Monographs*, No. 16 (1963).

Bloom, B.S. and O.L. Peterson, "End Results, Cost, and Productivity of Coronary Care Units," *The New England Journal of Medicine*, Vol. 288, No. 2: 72-78 (January 11, 1973).

Boulding, K.E., "The Concept of Need for Health Services," *Millbank Memorial Fund Quarterly*, pp. 202-223 (July 1966).

Center for Health Services Research and Development, American Medical Association, *The Profile of Medical Practice, 1972.* Chicago: American Medical Association, 1972.

Cohen, H., "Professional Licensure, Organizational Behavior, and the Public Interest," unpublished paper delivered at the Annual Meeting of the American Public Health Association. Atlantic City, New Jersey (November 14, 1972).

Crawford, R.L., and R.C. McCormack, "Reasons Physicians Leave Primary Practice." *Journal of Medical Education*, Vol. 46: 263-68 (April 1971).

Curtis, Elizabeth B., "Medication Errors Made by Patients," *Nursing Outlook*, Vol. 9, No. 5: 290-2 (May 1961).

David, W.D., "The Usefulness of Periodic Health Examinations," *Archives of Environmental Health*, Vol. 2, No. 3: 339-43 (March 1961).

Davis, Milton S., "Variations in Patients' Compliance with Doctors' Orders: Analysis of Congruence Between Survey Responses and Results of Empirical Investigations," *Journal of Medical Education*, Vol. 41, No. 11, Pt. 1: 1037 (November 1966).

Dean, Winston J., "Legal and Institutional Barriers to Health Manpower Productivity," unpublished staff paper, NCHSRD, HSMHA, DHEW (1972).

Densen, P.; E. Jones; E. Balamuth; and S. Shapiro, "Comparison of a Group Practice and a Self-Insurance Situation," *Hospitals*, Vol. 36: 63-68 (November 16, 1962).

————, "Prepaid Medical Care and Hospital Utilization in a Dual Choice Situation." *American Journal of Public Health*, Vol. 50: 1710-20 (November 1960).

Derbyshire, R.C., *Medical Licensure and Discipline in the United States.* Baltimore: The Johns Hopkins Press, 1969.

Donabedian, A., "An Evaluation of Prepaid Group Practice," *Inquiry*, Vol. 6: 3-27 (September 1969).

————, *A Review of Some Experiences with Prepaid Group Practice.* Ann Arbor: School of Public Health, University of Michigan, 1965.

Elliott, Robert V., "Demonstration and Evaluation of Computer-Assisted Analysis and Interpretation of the Electrocardiogram: A State-of-the-Art Report." Report submitted to Health Care Technology Division, NCHSRD, HSMHA, DHEW, under Contract No. HSM 110-69-414 (September 1972).

Fein, R., *The Doctor Shortage: An Economic Diagnosis.* Washington: The Brookings Institution, 1967.

Fein, R., and G.I. Weber, *Financing Medical Education.* New York: McGraw-Hill, 1971.

Feldstein, Martin S., "Hospital Cost Inflation: A Study of Non-Profit Price Dynamics," *American Economic Review*, Vol. 61: 853-72 (December 1971).

Forgotson, E.H., and Cook, J.L., "Innovations and Experiments in Uses of Health Manpower—The Effect of Licensure Laws." *Law and Contemporary Problems*, Vol. 32: 731-50 (Autumn 1967).

Franco, S.C. et al., "Periodic Health Examinations: A Long Term Study, 1949-59," *Journal of Occupational Medicine*, Vol. 3, No. 3, No. 1: 13-20 (January 1961).

Frech, H.E., "Occupational Licensure and Health Care: A Survey of the Literature," unpublished staff paper, NCHSRD, HSMHA, DHEW (1972).

Friedman, M., and Kuznets, S., *Income from Independent Professional Practice.* New York: National Bureau of Economic Research, 1945.

Fuchs, Victor R., and Kramer, Marcia J., *Determinants of Expenditures for Phsyicians' Services in the United States, 1948-1968.* Washington, D.C.: DHEW Publication No. (HSM) 73-3013, December 1972.

Garfield, Sidney R., "The Delivery of Medical Care," *Scientific American*, Vol. 222: 15-23 (April 1970).

Ginzberg, Eli, "Physician Shortage Reconsidered," *The New England Journal of Medicine*, Vol. 275: 85-7 (July 14, 1966).

Glazer, W.A., *Paying the Doctor*. Baltimore: The Johns Hopkins Press, 1970.

Golladay, Fredrick L., "Economic Implications of Patient Participation in Medical Care," unpublished issue paper submitted to Economic Analysis Branch, NCHSRD, HSMHA, DHEW (January 1973).

Golladay, Fredrick L.; M. Miller; and K.R. Smith, "An Analysis of Optimal Use of Inputs in the Production of Medical Services," *Journal of Human Resources*, Vol. 2: 208-50 (Spring 1972).

Golladay, Fredrick L.; Kenneth R. Smith; and Marianne Miller, "Allied Health Manpower Strategies: Estimates of the Potential Gains from Efficient Task Delegation." Research Reports Series No. 15, Health Economics Research Center, University of Wisconsin, (November 1971).

Graham, F.E., "Group Versus Solo Practice: Arguments and Evidence," *Inquiry*, Vol. 9: 49-60 (June 1972).

Greenfield, H.I., *Allied Health Manpower: Trends and Prospects*. New York: Columbia University Press, 1969.

Grimaldi, John V., "The Worth of Occupational Health Programs: A New Evaluation of Periodic Physical Examinations," *Journal of Occupational Medicine*, Vol. 7, No. 8: 365 (August 1965).

Gross, P.F., "Development and Implementation of Health Care Technology: The U.S. Experience," *Inquiry*, Vol. 9: 34-48 (June 1972).

Grossman, M., "On the Concept of Health Capital and the Demand for Health," *Journal of Political Economy*, Vol. 80: 223-55 (March/April 1972).

Hadley, Jack, "Background Paper for the Study of Physician Organization," unpublished paper, October 1972.

Held, P.J., "The Migration of 1955-1965 Graduates of American Medical Schools," unpublished Ph.D. dissertation, University of California, Berkeley, 1972.

Hershey, N., "An Alternative to Mandatory Licensure of Health Professionals," *Hospital Progress*, Vol. 50: 71-74 (March 1969).

Hughes, E.F.X.; V.R. Fuchs; J.E. Jacoby; and E.M. Lewit, "Surgical Workloads in a Community Practice," *Surgery*, Vol. 71: 315 (March 1972).

Hughes, E.F.X.; E.M. Lewit; R.N. Watkins; and R. Handschin, "Utilization of Surgical Manpower in a Prepaid Group Practice," Working Paper No. 19. New York: National Bureau of Economic Research, December 1973.

Human Resources Research Center, University of Southern California, "Analysis of the Utilization of Ancillary Personnel Using Production Functions," Working Paper, June 1972.

_____, "Direct Estimation of the Demand for Ancillary Personnel," Working Paper, March 1972a.

Human Resources Research Center, University of Southern California, "Estimation of Production Functions for Physicians' Services: Preliminary Results," Working Paper, March 1972b.

———, "The Specification and Estimation of Production Functions for Physicians' Services, Parts I and II," Working Paper, March 1971.

———, "Utilization of Ancillary Personnel by Physicians in Private Practice," Working Paper, March 1972c.

Intriligator, Michael D., and Barbara H. Kehrer, "A Simultaneous Equations Model of Ancillary Personnel Employed in Physicians' Offices," paper presented at the Econometric Society Meetings. Toronto, Canada (December 29, 1972).

James, Vernon L., and Warren E. Wheeler, "The Care-by-Patient Unit," *Pediatrics*, Vol. 43, No. 4: 488-494 (April 1964).

Kehrer, B.H., and H.W. Zaretsky, "A Preliminary Analysis of Allied Health Personnel in Primary Medical Practice," Working paper, Center for Health Services Research and Development, AMA, Chicago, 1972.

Kessel, R.A., "The AMA and the Supply of Physicians," *Law and Contemporary Problems*, Vol. 35: 267-83 (Spring 1970).

———, "Price Discrimination in Medicine," *Journal of Law and Economics*. Vol. 1: 20-53 (October 1958).

Kimbell, Larry J., and John H. Lorant, "Production Functions for Physicians' Services," Working paper submitted by Human Resources Research Center to Economic Analysis Branch, NCHSRD, HSMHA, DHEW, under Contract No. HSM 110-70-354 (December 1972).

Klarman, Herbert E., *The Economics of Health.* New York: Columbia University Press, 1965.

———, "Increase in the Cost of Physician and Hospital Services," *Inquiry*, Vol. 7: 22-36 (March 1970).

Kovner, J.W., "A Production Function for Outpatient Medical Facilities," unpublished Ph.D. dissertation, University of California, Los Angeles, 1968.

"The Legal Status of Physician's Assistants," *Hospital Progress*, pp. 44-50 (October 1972).

Linburn, G.E., "The Specter of Malpractice," *California Medicine*, pp. 50-4 (July 1969).

Mathis, R.L., "What Makes Doctors Want to Switch Careers," *Hospital Physician*, pp. 73-6 (December 1969).

Mechanic, David, and E.N. Volkart, "Stress, Illness Behavior, and the Sick Role," *American Sociological Review*, Vol. 26, No. 1: 51-58 (February 1961).

Mincer, J., "On-the-Job Training: Costs, Returns, and Some Implications," *Journal of Political Economy, Supplement*, pp. 50-79 (October 1962).

Monsma, G.N., "Marginal Revenue and the Demand for Physicians' Services," in *Empirical Studies in Health Economics*, edited by Herbert E. Klarman. Baltimore: The Johns Hopkins Press, 1970.

Moore, T.G., "The Purpose of Licensing," *The Journal of Law and Economics*, Vol. 4: 93-117 (October 1961).

Nelson, R.R., "Unanswered Questions About Miomedical Research: What Has it Done for Us, and How Did These Fine Things Come About?" unpublished working paper, July 1972.

Newhouse, J.P., "The Economics of Group Practice," *Journal of Human Resources*, Vol. 8: 37-56 (Winter 1973).

Owens, A., "How Many Doctors Are Really Working at Full Capacity?" *Medical Economics*, pp. 85-93 (January 18, 1971).

Pauly, M., "Efficiency, Incentives and Reimbursement for Health Care," *Inquiry*, Vol. 7: 114-31 (March 1970).

Peterson, O.S.; F.J. Lyden; H.J. Geiger; and T. Colton, "Appraisal of Medical Students' Abilities as Related to Training and Careers after Graduation," *New England Journal of Medicine*, Vol. 289: 1174-82 (1963).

Pragoff, Hale, "Adjustment of Tuberculosis Patients One Year After Hospital Discharge," *Public Health Reports*, Vol. 77, No. 8: 671-9 (August 1962).

Preston, D.F., and F.L. Miller, "The Tuberculous Outpatient's Defection from Therapy," *American Journal of the Medical Sciences*, Vol. 247, No. 1: 21-25 (January 1964).

"Progress Report on Departmental Actions and Recommendations in the *Report on Licensure and Related Health Personnel Credentialing*." Rockville, Md.: NCHSRD, unpublished staff paper, 1972.

Rafferty, J.A., "Patterns of Hospital Use: An Analysis of Short-Run Variation," *Journal of Political Economy*, Vol. 79: 154-65 (January/February 1971).

Rayack, E., *Professional Power and American Medicine: The Economics of the American Medical Association*. New York: World, 1967.

Reder, M.W., "Some Problems in the Measurement of Productivity in the Medical Care University," in *Production and Productivity in the Service Industries*, edited by Victor R. Fuchs. New York: Columbia University Press, 1969.

Reiffen, Barney and Anthony Komaroff, "The Ambulatory Care Project, ACS-II Evaluation Plan," submitted to Health Care Technology Division, NCHSR, HRA, DHEW under Contract No. HSM 110-73-335, December 1972.

Reinhardt, U.E., "An Economic Analysis of Physicians' Practices," unpublished Ph.D. dissertation, Yale University, 1970.

_____ , "A Production Function for Physicians' Services," *The Review of Economics and Statistics*, Vol. 54: 55-66 (February 1972).

Reinhardt, U.E., and Donald E. Yett, "Physician Production Functions Under Varying Practice Arrangements," Technical Paper Series No. 1, Community Profile Data Center, HSMHA, DHEW (January 1971).

"Report of the Federal Council for Science and Technology, Committee on Automation Opportunities in the Service Areas, Panel on Health Services," unpublished, Washington, D.C. (May 1972).

Report on Licensure and Related Health Personnel Credentialing, Department of

Health, Education, and Welfare. Washington, D.C.: U.S. Government Printing Office, 1971.

Report of the National Advisory Commission on Health Manpower. Washington, D.C.: U.S. Government Printing Office, 1967.

Report of the President's Commission on Malpractice, Washington, D.C.: U.S. Government Printing Office, January 1973.

Riddick, F.A., et al., "Use of Allied Health Professionals in Internists' Offices," *Archives of Internal Medicine*, Vol. 127: 924-31 (May 1971).

Robbins, A., "Allied Health Manpower," *Inquiry*, Vol. 7: 55-61 (March 1970).

Roemer, Milton I., "Hospital Utilization and the Supply of Physicians," *Journal of the American Medical Association*, Vol. 178: 125-29 (December 9, 1961).

Rosenberg, Stanley G., "Patient Education Leads to Better Care for Heart Patients," *HSMHA Health Reports*, Vol. 86, No. 9: 793-802 (September 1971).

Scheffler, Richard M., "Productivity and Economies of Scale in Medical Practice," issue paper submitted to Economics Analysis Branch, NCHSRD, HSMHA, DHEW (September 1972).

Scheffler, Richard M., and D. Stinson, "An Analysis of the Supply of Physicians' Assistants," working paper, Health Services Research Center, University of North Carolina, 1972.

Schwartz, Doris, et al., "Medication Errors Made by Elderly Chronically Ill Patients," *American Journal of Public Health*, Vol. 52, No. 12: 2018-29 (December 1962).

Shephard, R.W., *Therapy of Cost and Production Functions.* Princeton, N.J.: Princeton University Press, 1970.

Simonds, Scott K., "Motivation and Health Insurance," in *Proceedings of Second National Conference on Health Education.* Chicago: American Medical Association, 1966.

Sloan, F.A., "Economic Models of Physician Supply," unpublished Ph.D. dissertation, Harvard University, 1968.

———, "Effects of Incentives on Physician Practice Performance," issue paper submitted to Economic Analysis Branch, NCHSRD, HSMHA, DHEW (January 1973a).

———, *Supply Responses of Young Physicians: An Analysis of Physicians in Residency Programs.* Santa Monica, Cal.: Rand Corporation R-1131-OEO, 1973b.

Taylor, V., and J. Newhouse, *Ambulatory Care at the Good Samaritan Medical Center.* Santa Monica, Cal.: Rand Corporation RM-6342, 1970.

Theodore, C.N.; G.E. Sutter; and J.N. Haug, *Medical School Alumni.* Chicago: American Medical Association, 1967.

Thomas, L., "Notes of a Biology Watcher; The Technology of Medicine," *The New England Journal of Medicine*, pp. 1366-68 (December 9, 1971).

Ulrich, Marian R., and Kenneth M. Kelley, "Patient Care Includes Teaching:

Health Education Department Coordinates Multidisciplinary Programs," *Hospitals*, Vol. 46: 59-65 (April 1972).

Wade, L. et al., "Are Periodic Health Examinations Worthwhile?" *Annals of Internal Medicine*, Vol. 56, No. 1: 81-93 (January 1962).

Waxman, Bruce, and Maxine Rockoff, "Technology and Productivity, and their Relationship to New Organizational Schemes for Health Care Delivery," unpublished staff paper, Health Care Technology Division, NCHSRD, HSMHA, DHEW (1972).

Weinerman, R., "Problems and Perspectives in Group Practice," *Group Practice*, Vol. 18: 27-33 (April 1969).

Weisbrod, B., "Costs and Benefits of Medical Research: A Case Study of Poliomyelitis," *Journal of Political Economy*, Vol. 79: 527-44 (May/June 1971).

Weiss, J.H., "The Changing Structure of Health Manpower," unpublished Ph.D. dissertation, Harvard University, 1966.

Yankauer, A.; J.P. Connelly; and J.J. Feldman, "Task Performance and Task Delegation in Pediatric Office Practice," *American Journal of Public Health*, Vol. 59: 1104-11 (July 1969).

————, "Pediatric Practice in the United States, with Special Attention to Utilization of Allied Health Worker Services," *Pediatrics*, Vol. 45: 521-51 (March 1970a).

————, "Physician Productivity in the Delivery of Ambulatory Care: Some Findings from a Survey of Pediatricians," *Medical Care*, Vol. 8: 35-46 (January/February 1970b).

Yett, D.E., "An Evaluation of Alternative Methods of Estimating Physician's Expenses Relative to Output," *Inquiry*, Vol. 4: 3-27 (March 1967).

Yett, D.E., and F.A. Sloan, "Analysis of Migration Patterns of Recent Medical School Graduates." Rockville, Md.: NCHSRD, 1972.

Index

Index

Abramowitz: dental care, Department of Indian Health, 110-111

Accreditation: definition of, Dean, 182

Acquired regulation theory: licensure, 120

Activities, potential: computerization, 165-166

Activity analysis: approach to ambulatory care, Smith, Miller, & Golladay, 20; Zeckhauser and Eliastam, Physicians' Assistants use, 21

Activity analysis techniques: ancillary substitution, Golladay, Smith, and Miller, 158-159

"Adverse selection problem": cost and productivity, 66

Aide input: optimum level, 18; vs physician input, 7

Aide utilization by physicians, 18-19

Aides: increased output using, Reinhardt, 23

Aiken: nursing in individual health care instruction, 92

Allied health occupations, licensed, 123

Allied health personnel: AMA educational standards, Robbins, 126-127; education program categories, 126-127; "institutional licensure", 132; labor market for, research needed, 189; primary care practices, 159

"Allied Health Workers" traditional (AHWs): categories, by education, 14; categories by use, 14-15; assistants, 14; definition of health practitioners, 24; increased need due to PNPs, 28; output, case-mix variation, 24; physicians and patient visits, 26; professionals, 14; relation to number of aides, 22-23; role and function, 22-23; role of, empirical studies, 23-24; role of physician extenders, 24; task delegation, 22-23; technicians, 14

Allocation of resources: health services, 143

Alternative reimbursement schemes: incentives, 178; incentives, Sloan, 178; productivity, 178

Ambulatory care: activity analysis approach, Smith, Miller, and Golladay, 20; manpower substitution, 3; output definition, 11-12; productive factors, 13-14

Ambulatory care output: classification of provider facilities, 12; definition of, 12

Ambulatory care production: definition of "technical processes", 20; direct observation, 31-32; input definitions and measurements, 13-14; research needed, 30; time and motion studies, 30

Amendment to Immigration Act: foreign physicians, immigration, 131

American Cancer Society: health care utilization, in cancer detection, 90

American Medical Association, AMA: educational standards, allied health personnel, Robbins, 126-127; National Mean charges, 67; opposition to foreign physicians, 131; paramedical personnel, Rayack, 123; variation in costs per patient visit, 67

AMA and AHA: paramedical personnel licensing, 128

AMA National Survey: group vs solo practice, patient visits, 48

American-trained physicians: licensing mechanism, 122

Analyses of production framework: 4

Ancillaries: greater use of, 160-164; malpractice insurance premiums, Intriligator and Kehrer, 161; pediatricians' task delegation, 159; President's Commission on Malpractice, 161; use of productivity gains, Bailey, 164-165

Ancillary marginal productivity: physician shortage, 159

Ancillary personnel: input substitution questions, 157; input-output analysis, research needed, 189; licensure law restrictions, 183; production functions, research needed, 189; productivity and group size, 174, 176; solo physicians, 157; task delegation, research needed, 189

Ancillary services: economies of scale, 173

Ancillary substitution: activity analysis techniques, Golladay, Smith, and Miller, 158-159; productivity increase, 158-160; Reinhardt, 154

Ancillary substitution, production function technique: Bailey, 157; Kehrer and Zaretsky, 157; Kimbell and Lorant, 157; Reinhardt, 157; Reinhardt and Yett, 157

Ancillary utilization: demand pressures, 159; excess demand, Riddick et al., 186; excess demand, Yankauer et al., 186; interstate licensure variations, research needed, 193; physician services, excess demand, research needed, 189; productivity gains, 160

Annual gross billings: as output index, 16

"Anxiety-driven" system: health care system, 148

Arnold: time saved by use of dental auxiliaries, 112

Automated medical history results: Waxman and Rockoff, 167

Auxiliaries, utilization of: Riddick et al., 159; Yankauer, Connelly, and Feldman, 159

Auxiliary health manpower: in output definition, 14

Auxiliary health personnel, value of: prior research, 21-22

Auxiliary personnel: equivalency qualifications, 183; in output definition, 14; input "support", 21; physician nonutilization of Human Resources Research Center, 160

Average production function, 10

Average productivity, 6

Bailey: average physician productivity, 46; constant returns to scale, 46; economies of scale, 173; economies of scale in group vs solo practices, 45; production function techniques, ancillary substitution, 157; productivity by group practice size, 70; productivity studies,

207

Bailey (cont.)
  production function, 43-44; use of productivity gains from ancillaries, 164-165
Baird et al.: Canadian military program, dental "clinical technicians", 111
Balfe and McNamara: varying share of net income, income distribution, 65
Barnett: computer applications in medicine, 165
Benefits, potential: computerization, 165-166
Berkeley Scientific Laboratories: computerization, diagnosis, 166
Berki: productivity and group practice size, 174, 176
Berkowitz: patient noncompliance, physicians' perceptions of, 88
Bharara: smallpox innoculation education, 90
Biomedical advances: death rates, 154; productivity growth, Fuchs and Kramer, 153-154
Black medical schools, 124, 125
Blackwell: patient sick role, 88; "sick role" and seeking medical care, 169
Bloomgarden: Jewish medical students, proportion of, 125
Boaz, studies: production function estimates, 16
Boulding: health and disease, adaptive concepts, 188
Brown: dental practitioners and dental auxiliaries, 114

California Relative Value Scale (CRVS): output weights, 148; surgery, Hughes et al., 174
Cancer detection: health care utilization in, American Cancer Society, 90; health care utilization in, Kegeles et al., 90; health care utilization in, Miyaska, 90
Capital: equipment utilization studies, 196, notes; input, clinics studies, 32-33, notes; noncomputer based, potential, research needed, 190; privately vs publically developed, diffusion patterns, research needed, 190
Capital purchasing: demand pressures, research needed, 190; reimbursement schemes, research needed, 190
Capital substitution: economic feasibility of, research needed, 189; health manpower, productivity, 165-168; incentives for, research needed, 190; input substitution, 155; output, research needed, 190; production function inputs, 165; research needed, 168
Capitation arrangements: income incentives, 60
Capitation equations: equal income sharing, 61; individual physician output, 61; physician income, 61
Capitation practices: effects on incentive, 62; group demand schedule, 62
Capitation reimbursement: incentives, 155-156
Capitation reimbursement scheme, 179
Care-by-parent: University of Kentucky Medical Center, 89-90
Case-mix: demand pressures, Rafferty, 159; output measurement, 50, notes; output measurement, Feldstein, 50, notes
Case-mix variation: AHWs output, 24; cost and

productivity, 67
Causes and solutions: patient noncompliance, 87-88
Certification: alternative to licensure, 121; alternative to licensure, Friedman, 132; definition of, Dean, 182
Charges, National mean: AMA, 67
Charles F. Miller Hospital program: diabetes self-care, 89
Chemotherapy: patient noncompliance, 87
Child Health Associate: Physician's Assistant, 24
Chiropractors, increase of licensure, 123
Chronic disease protocol: diabetes clinic, 167; Reiffen and Komaroff, 167
Chronic problems: cost-effective patient participation: 93, 94
Clinics: as opposed to small practice in flexibility of medical care services, 29; capital input studies, 32-33, notes; Kovner studies, 32-33, notes
Cobb, Douglas: modified production function form, 17; production function form, 172
Coefficients, input: combinations of, 5, 6
Coefficients, input-output, 5, 6; efficiency estimate, 9; estimation of, 9; identification of range, 9
Community size reallocation: increased physician productivity, 186
Communications technologies: in health care, Waxman and Rockoff, 165
Compensation: of group practice management, 63-64
Compensation, varying share: group size, 64-65
Competency, maintenance of needed: licensing, Dean, 183
Competition, health occupation: Greenfield, 127-128; licensure, 128
Competition, medical: prevention of Friedman, 126-127; Kessel, 126-127; Rayack, 126-127
Competition, price discrimination: licensure, 135, notes
Competition, professional: Greenfield, 136
Compliance: patient, Davis, 87-88; reasons for patient noncompliance, research needed, 191
Comprehensive Health Insurance Plan: Health Maintenance Organization (HMO), xiv
Comprehensive Health Manpower Strategy: DHEW, xiii
Comprehensive prepaid medical group ("CPMG"), 42; value of inputs, 42
Computer application in medicine: Barnett, 165
Computer-assisted electrocardiogram: analysis, Elliot, 166; physician time saved, 167
Computer-based practices: health services, 165-168
Computerization: chemistry laboratories, Waxman and Rockoff, 166; data analysis, 166; diagnosis, Berkeley Scientific Laboratories, 166; diagnosis, economic feasibility, 166; multiphasic screening, Garfield, 168; potential activities, 165-166; potential benefits, 165-166; operating costs reduced, 166; physician time saved, 165-166
"Conditions managed" as output index, 13

Constant average costs: no economies of scale, 41

Constant: elasticity-of-substitution (CES) production function, 21-22

Constant returns to scale: Bailey, 46; production function, 41

Consumer expenditures on dental care: dental output measurement, 109-110

Continuous production functions: algebraic form discussed, 11; data collection and interpretation, 16; empirical estimates, 16-17; estimates of, 10; estimates of, manpower substitution, 15; estimation of various forms, 30; inputs, 16; research needed, 30; unit of analysis, 16

Controversy over licensure, 119-120

"Cost and insurance": approach to productivity, Reder, 42

Cost and productivity: "adverse selection problem", 66; case-mix variation, 67; effects of income sharing, 57; in alternative practice setting, 66-67; incentive structure difficulties, 66; incentives, cost-sharing vs non-cost-sharing, 61; licensure reform, 133

Cost benefit analysis research strategy: Weisbrod, 194

Cost curve, average: Newhouse, 47

Cost-effective modes, patient participation: research needed, 191

Cost-effective patient education, 95; research needed, 191

Cost-effective patient participation, 168; chronic problems, 93, 94; in health maintenance, 94; short-term episodic problems, 93

Cost-effective programs: patient self-care, 89

Cost equations: equal shares cost-sharing, 57; physicians' personal cost, 58

Cost function, 55; average, economies of scale, Newhouse, 173-174; economies of scale, 47, 48; estimation, economies of scale, Yett, 175-177; optimum practice size, Shephard, 172

Cost (income) sharing arrangements: revenue, 54,55

Cost-sharing: expense function, 48; fixed and/or variable, 54, 55; group practice, 54, 55; group practice, Newhouse, 53; group practice management, 63; group practice size, 56-67; marginal income gain, 56-57; physician incentive, 56-57; physician income, 56

Cost-sharing and income-cost-sharing: effects on group practice, 180

Cost-sharing arrangements: group vs solo practice, 46, 47

Cost-sharing effects: revenue, 53-54

Cost-sharing, equal shares: cost equations, 57; revenue, 57

Cost-sharing, revenue: unequal shares, equation, 59; unequal shares, incentives, 60

Cost-sharing vs non-cost-sharing: cost and productivity incentives, 61

Cost, marginal: imputed physician cost, 80, note; marginal revenue, 80, note

Cost of hospitalization: Feldstein, 185

Cost parameters: group practice size, 61

Cost of physicians: nonlicensed medical personnel, 123

Cost of productivity: Donabedian, 49

Cost per visit: earnings loss, 59

Cost reduction incentive, marginal, nonphysician, 58

Cost reductions: patient education, 93

Costs: imputed physician and marginal, 80, note; licensure effects, 182; patient education, 93; patient participation, 93; preventive care, David, 168-169; preventive care, Grinaldi, 168-169

Costs, average, increasing: diseconomies of scale, 41

Costs, average, of production: economies of scale, 41

Costs, increasing, medical care, xiii

Costs, operating, reduced: computerization, 166

Costs, overhead, per patient visit: Taylor and Newhouse, 177

Costs and returns: individual group practice member, 53

Costs per patient visit, variations in: American Medical Association, 67; Newhouse, 67; private practice vs outpatient clinics, 67; Sloan, 67; Taylor and Newhouse, 67

Crawford and McCormack: physician reallocation studies, 186

Creighton: smallpox innoculation education, 90

Creighton and Gabrielle: group teaching, learning problems, 92

Cross and Parsons: nursing in individual health care instruction, 92

Cross sectional analysis: licensure, 134

Curtis: patient compliance, elderly, 169; patient noncompliance, 87

Data analysis: computerization, 166

Data collection and interpretation: continuous production functions, 16; description of task delegation, 15

David: preventive care, 87; preventive care, costs, 168-169

Davis: patient compliance, 87-88

Dean: definition of accreditation, 182; definition of certification, 182; definition of licensure, 182; licensing, equivalency qualifications, 183; maintenance of competency needed, licensing, 183; new health manpower categories, licensing, 182

Death rates: biomedical advances, 154

Decision-making: in various practice modes, research needed, 77, 79; group practice management surveys, 63; group vs individual, 76

Delivery system: manpower substitution, 29-30

Demand conditions: "real" output, 186; real productivity, 186

Demand curve: equation, 55; physicians', 55

Demand, excess: ancillary utilization, Riddick et al., 186; ancillary utilization, Yankauer et al., 186; physician incentive, 186; physician services, ancillary utilization, research needed, 189

Demand of hospitalization and cases treated: Rafferty, 185-186

Demand pressures: ancillary utilization, 159; capital purchasing, research needed, 190; case-mix, Rafferty, 159

Dental assistants: see also "dental therapists"

Dental assistants: dental health teams, Department of Indian Health, 110-111; limits and training of, Johnson and Bernstein, 113-114; Lotzkar et al. study, 110; Louisville, Ky. Division of Mental Health Study, 110; use of and time saved, 112

Dental auxiliaries: see also dental assistants

Dental auxiliaries: see also "expanded function auxiliaries" (EFAs)

Dental auxiliaries: attitudes toward, dental practitioners, 114; Canadian study, Hall, 115, notes; defined by state dental licensing boards, 113; dental output, 109-110; dental practices act, Minnesota, 115-116, notes; dentist-patient relationships, 114; expanded function, 112; expanded use of, World Health Organization advice, 112; increased dental output, 112-113; increased productivity, 108; restraints on, dental practice acts, 113; restraints on use, 113; time saved by use of, Arnold, 112; use of, dental productivity, 109

Dental auxiliaries and dental practitioners, Brown, 114

Dental care: consumer expenditures on, dental output measurement, 109-110; Department of Indian Health, Abramowitz, 110-111; supply of, 107

Dental "clinical technicians": Canadian military program, Baird et al., 111; dental hygienists, 111; individualized training, 111; effect on dental productivity, 115, notes

Dental health teams: Department of Indian Health dental assistants, 110-111

Dental hygienists: dental "clinical technicians", 111; dental practice acts, 113; increasing use, 112; licensure restrictions, 130

Dental licensing: State dental examinating (licensing) boards, 113

Dental manpower shortage: foreign countries, 112

Dental nurse program, New Zealand: Walsh, 112

Dental output: dental auxiliaries, 109-110; increased by dental auxiliaries, 112-113; increased, measures of, 108; limited by dental practice acts, 113; production function, 115, notes; research needed, 114

Dental output mixes, dentists and auxiliaries: research needed, 114

Dental output measurement: consumer expenditures on dental care, 109-110; dental sector, 114; gross incomes of dentists, 109-110; patient visits, 109-110; "procedures completed per day", 110

Dental practice acts: dental hygienists, 113; dental output, limited by, 113; Minnesota-dental auxiliaries, 115-116, notes; restraints on dental auxiliaries, 113

Dental practitioners: attitudes toward, dental auxiliaries, 114

Dental practitioners and dental auxiliaries: Brown, 114

Dental productivity: dental equipment effect on, 115, notes; increase, "expanded function auxiliaries" (EFAs), 114; nonlabor inputs and technical change, 114; technical change over time, Maurizi, 115, notes; use of dental auxiliaries, 109

Dental schools: supply and demand, 107-108

Dental sector: output measurement, dental, 114

Dental services: inputs, 108; production of, 108; public, New Zealand-type nurses, 112

Dental "technicians": see also dental "clinical technicians"

Dental "technicians": dentists' use of time, 112; efficiency, Ludwig, 111; increased productivity, 111-112; quality of work, Ludwig, 111; training, Ludwig, 111

Dental therapists: see also "technotherapists"

Dental therapists: Hammons, 110; tasks performed, 110

Dentist: patient relationships, dental auxiliaries, 114

Dentist and physician mobility: licensure effects, 182

Dentistry: included in NHI plan, xv; manpower productivity, 107; operative, "technotherapists", 111; technology of, 108

Dentists: foreign-trained, 107

Dentists: use of time, dental technicians, 112

Dentists and auxiliaries: dental output mixes, research needed, 114

Department of Health, Education and Welfare (DHEW): comprehensive health manpower strategy, xiii; licensure reforms experiments, 133; licensure report, jurisdictional restrictionism, 128

Department of Indian Health: dental care, Abramowitz, 110-111; dental health teams, dental assistants, 110-111

Derbyshire: foreign medical students, state licensure examinations, 132; foreign-trained health workers, mobility, 130

Deterrent to specific practice mode choices, 76, 78

Diabetes clinic: chronic disease protocol, 167

Diffusion patterns: privately vs publically developed capital, research needed, 190

Direct observation: ambulatory care production, 31-32

Discrimination: against foreign medical graduates, 130-132; Jewish physicians, Kessel, 124-125, 126; medical schools, 123-126

"Discrimination index": lack of efficiency index, 32

Disease treatment histories: research strategy, 194

Diseases, undetected disabling: Franco et al., 168-169; Wade et al., 168-169

Diseconomies of scale-increasing average costs, 41

Doctor "shortage": demand for physicians, 3; national health insurance increased, 3
Donabedian: group vs solo practice, patient visits, 48; productivity cost, 49
Dual cost function: production function, 41

Earnings loss: cost per visit, 59
Economic analysis of health maintenance: research needed, 191
Economic analysis of patient participation: research needed, 191
Economic cost: physician reallocation, Sloan, 186
Economic efficiency: alternative modes of health care, 86; health care, Health Plan of Greater New York, 86; health care, Kaiser-Permanente system, 86; health services, research needed, 143; periodic examinations, 87; various practice modes, Frech and Ginsburg, 80, note
Economic feasibility: capital substitution, research needed, 189; computerization, diagnosis, 166; input substitution, 155
Economic implications: of patient education, 93; of patient participation in health care, 94
Economic incentives: manpower substitution, 30
Economically efficient combinations: of production processes, 32, notes; of technical substitution, 32, notes
Economically optimal characterization of production process, 5-6
The Economics of Health, Klarman: health economics research, 152
Economics research, health: data scarcity, 152; empirical, 152
Economies of scale: ancillary services, 173; average cost function, Newhouse, 173-174; average costs of production, 41; Bailey, 173; Cobb-Douglas form, Kimbell and Lorant, 172; cost function estimation, Yett, 175-177; cost functions, 47, 48; definition framework, 39; group and solo practices comparison, 45-46; group practice, 29, 170-ff; group practice, production function, 171; group practice size, 173; group vs solo practices, Bailey, 45; group vs solo practices, Newhouse, 45; incentives, Newhouse, 173; income, 173; Kovner, 48; output, 47; output measurement, 46; production function, 171; productivity, 45-46; productivity, conceptual difficulties, 172; productivity, Kovner, 45-46; productivity, Reinhardt, 45-46; solo practice, 29; studied separately from production functions, 41-42; workweek, 173; Yett, 47
Economies of scale, no, constant average costs, 41
Economies of scale or production function: to study group and solo practices, 41-42
Education, patient: see patient education
Education, smallpox innoculation: Bharara, 90; Creighton, 90
Education, target population: smallpox innoculation studies, 90

Education and training: licensure requirements, 182-183
Education and training, medical: impact of, research needed, 193-194
Education of health care workers, 126-127
Education program categories: allied health personnel, 126-127
Education provided by group practice: research needed, 193
Educational Council for Foreign Medical Graduates (ECFMG), 130-131
Educational Council for Foreign Medical Graduates exam foreign medical students, licensure, 130-131; passing rates, Stevens and Vermeulen, 131
Educational standards: AMA, allied health personnel, Robbins, 126-127
Educational structure: manpower quality changes, 156
Efficiency, economic: see economic efficiency
Elliot: computer-assisted electrocardiogram analysis, 166
Empirical estimates: continuous production functions, 16-17
Endorsement-licensure, 136
Equal income-sharing: capitation equation, 61; effects on incentive, 62
Equal income-sharing group incentives: individual physician output, 59
Equal shares cost-sharing: cost equations, 57; revenue, 57
Equivalency and proficiency procedures needed: licensure, 183
Equivalency qualifications: auxiliary personnel, 183; licensing, Dean, 183
"Expanded function auxiliaries" (EFAs) see also dental auxiliaries
"Expanded function auxiliaries (EFAs): dental productivity, 110; New Zealand program, 110
Expense function: cost-sharing, 48
Expenses per visit: by type of practice, 68-69; practice, 67

Family nurse practitioners: improved use of, 23; Physicians' Assistant, 24
Federal role: medical services, 53
Fee-for-service physicians, 54
Fee-for-service practices: physician income and incentive, 70; productivity, 70
Fee-for-service reimbursement scheme, 178-179; incentives, Monsma, 178; incentives for overdoctoring, Ginsberg, 155
Fee-for-service vs salaried practice: output, 71-72
Fee-setting practices, group: Rorem, 80-81
Feldman: patient knowledge of health care, 90
Feldstein: case-mix as output measurement, 50, notes; cost of hospitalization, 185; Reder's productivity measurements, 42
Financial security vs income potential, 72, 77
Flexner Report, 1910: licensing, 124
Formal patient instruction methods: Young, 91
Foreign citizens: specialty boards, 129

Foreign countries: dental manpower shortage, 112

Foreign medical graduates: discrimination against, 130-132; ECFMG exam, licensure, 130-131; licensure barriers, 184

Foreign medical students: state licensure examinations, Derbyshire, 132; Stevens and Vermeulen, law suit at Guadalajara U, 132

Foreign physicians: amendment to Immigration Act, 131; AMA opposition to, 131; labor department immigration rules, 131-132

Foreign-trained dentists, 107

Foreign-trained health workers: licensure restrictions, 130; mobility, Derbyshire, 130

Foreign-trained medical graduates: House of Representatives Subcommittee of the Committee on the Judiciary, 131

Foreign-trained medical personnel restrictions: Stevens and Vermeulen, 131

Forgotson and Cook, paramedical personnel licensing, 128

Fractionation: definition of, Klarman, 195, notes

Franco et al.: preventive care, 86-87; undetected disabling diseases, 168-169

Frech: licensure effects, productivity, 182

Frech and Ginsburg: economic efficiency of various practice modes, 80, note

Friedman: certification system as licensure alternative, 132

Fuchs and Kramer: biomedical advances, productivity growth, 153-154

Gains in productivity, 6

Garfield: multiphasic screening, computerization, 168

Gellhorn: licensure in general, 135, notes

General practitioners: hospital access restrictions, 129

General practitioners vs specialists: Rayack, 129

Geographical location: physician choice of, Yett and Sloan, 187

Geographical reallocation: increased physician productivity, 186

Geographical restrictions: licensure, 129-130

Ginzberg: fee-for-service reimbursement scheme, incentives for overdoctoring, 155

Goldberg: advantages of salaried practice, 73; Jews admitted to medical schools, 124-125, 126

Golladay: formal patient education, 170; informal and individual patient education, 170; patient involvement in medical care, 168; patient knowledge and self-care, 170; preventive care, innoculations, 168-169

Golladay, Smith, and Miller: activity analysis techniques, ancillary substitution, 158-159

Greenfield: health occupation competition, 127-128; professional competition, 136

Grinaldi: preventive care, 87; preventive care costs, 168-169

Group and solo practices: economies of scale comparison, 45-46; inputs and maximum output, 39; studied by economics of scale or production function, 41-42

Group decision-making: structure of incentives, research needed, 192

Group demand schedule: capitation practices, 62; prepayment retainer practices, 181

Group fee-setting practices: Rorem, 80-81

Group manager: effect on productivity, 49

Group partnerships: initial incomes, Jeffers, 81; initial incomes, *Medical Economics*, 81

Group-partnership vs solo practice: income differences, 71, 73, 74-75

Group practice, xv; cost-sharing, 54, 55; cost sharing, Newhouse, 53; economies of scale, 29, 170-ff; economies of scale, production function, 171; education provided by, research needed, 193; effects on cost-sharing and income-cost-sharing, 180; income distribution methods, 65; multispecialty, research needed, 49-50; output and physician income, 81; physician productivity, 53; price setting, 58; production function, 171; production function output, returns to scale, 40; productivity, 70; productivity gains from organizational changes, 155-156

Group practice, individual member: cost and returns, 53; inherent incentives effects, 53; profit and income distribution, 63-64; income equations, 58

Group practice management, 54; compensation of, 63-64; cost-sharing, 63; decision-making surveys, 63

Group practice managers: incentives, 181; reimbursement scheme preferences, 181; research needed, 192

Group practice physician: effect of income sharing on productivity, 49; multispecialty, 44; single-specialty, 44

Group practice plans, prepaid, 196, notes

Group practice size: cost parameters, 61; cost-sharing, 56-57; economies of scale, 173; effect on productivity, 173; output, 70; productivity, ancillary personnel, 174, 176; productivity, Bailey, 70; productivity, Berki, 174, 176; productivity, Kovner, 173; productivity, Yankauer et al., 70, 174-175; structure of incentives, research needed, 192

Group production function: output, returns to scale, 40

Group size: effect on value of leisure, 66; varying share compensation, 64-65

Group size and output: income (revenue-cost) sharing groups, 62

Group teaching: learning problems, Creighton and Gabrielle, 92; patient education, 91-92

Group vs individual decision-making, 76

Group vs solo practice: cost sharing arrangements, 46, 47; hours and weeks worked, 70-71; income considerations, 72, 77; median net incomes, 47; office visits, 46; output, 70; patient visits, AMA National Survey, 48; patient visits, Donabedian, 48; patient visits, *Medical Economics* Survey, 48; productivity, 70, 170ff; productivity, Reinhardt, 44; pro-

Group vs solo practice (cont.)
ductivity difference, 48; Scheffler, 170;
Sloan, 170; weeks worked, *Medical Economics*, 71, 72; weeks worked, Owens, 71,
72; workweeks, 70, 71
Guadalajara U., law suit: foreign medical students, Stevens and Vermeulen, 132

Hall: dental auxiliaries, Canadian study, 115,
notes
Hallburg: patient instruction, individual, 91
Hammons: "dental therapists", 110
Health and disease, adaptive concepts: Boulding, 188
Health care: communications technology, Waxman and Rockoff, 165; economic efficiency
of, Health Plan of Greater New York, 86;
economic efficiency of, Kaiser-Permanente
System, 86; economic efficiency of alternative modes, 86; effects on health status, 86;
Health Plan of Greater New York, 86; individual instruction, 92; instruction with treatment, 92; Kaiser-Permanente System, 86;
market value as quality index, 149-150; nursing in individual instruction, Aiken, 92; nursing in individual instruction, Cross and Parsons, 92; occupational licensure, 119; office
visit instruction, Renner, 92; patient knowledge of, 90; patient knowledge of, Kirscht et
al., 90; patient participation, economic implications, 94; patient participation, research
needed, 94; patient participation in, behavior
change, research needed, 190-192; patient
role in, 92; preventive, presumed value, 92;
quality and limits, 148-151; quality index,
relative input prices, 150; quality of, prices,
150-151; utilization in cancer detection,
A.C.S., 90; utilization in cancer detection,
Kegeles et al., 90; utilization in cancer detection, Miyaska, 90; value judgments, quality, 149-151; variables in patient willingness
to utilize, 89
Health care institutions: "institutional licensure", 132
Health care workers: education of, 126-127
Health care providers: definition of homogeneity in, 14
Health care system: as "anxiety-driven" system,
148; patient role in utilization of, 88; utilization of, patient seeking intervention, 88
Health economics research: data scarcity, 152;
empirical, 152; Klarman, *The Economics of
Health*, 152
Health education: preventive, 87-89
Health Education Monograph: patient education, 91
Health maintenance: cost-effective patient participation, 94; economic analysis of, research
needed, 191; research needed, 94
Health Maintenance Organizations (HMOs),
49-50; comprehensive health insurance plan,
xiv; issues raised, 39
Health manpower: effects of technical change
on quality, research needed, 194; flexibility

of medical care services, 29; full utilization,
29; input-output measurement, 145-146;
licensing mechanism, 122; licensure barriers
to utilization, 184; new categories, licensing,
Dean, 182; occupational licensure, 119; quality of care and skill, 148-151; quality of new,
research needed, 193-194; total productivity,
145
Health manpower productivity: capital substitution, 165-168; input-output relationship,
143
Health manpower substitution: input-output,
Weiss, 154; productivity growth, 154-155
Health occupations, competition: Greenfield,
127-128; licensure, 128
Health personnel: low-skilled, Weiss, 123
Health Plan of Greater New York: economic
efficiency of health care, 86; health care, 86
Health practitioners: definition of, 24; impact
in pediatric office, 28
Health production: issues in defining output,
146-147
Health profession supply: licensure restriction
of, 122
Health professionals, selection of: manpower
quality changes, 156
Health services: allocation of resources, 143;
computer-based practices, 165-168; definition
of, 144; economic efficiency of research
needed, 143; input categories, 144; input-output variables, 145-146; inputs, production
function, 144-145; production function,
idealized, 146
Health services productivity: effect of patient
ignorance, 147; insurance effect on price index, 147; licensure, 119; production function, 144
Health status: effects of health care on, 86
Heart disease education: patient self-care,
Rosenberg, 170
Held: physician migratory behavior, 187
Hershey: "institutional licensure" proposal,
132; paramedical personnel licensing, 128
Hessel and Haggerty: telephone contact time,
physicians and PNP, 28
HEW report: licensure, 126-127
Homogeneity: definition of, health care providers, 14
Hospital Physician survey: practice mode, physician preference, 72, 76
Hospital physicians: productivity, 175, 176
Hours and weeks worked: group vs solo practice, 70-71
House of Representatives Subcommittee of the
Committee on the Judiciary: foreign-trained
medical graduates, 131
Hughes: relative value scales as output weights,
148
Hughes et al.: California Relative Value Scale,
surgery, 174
Human Resources Research Center: physicians'
nonutilization of auxiliary personnel, 160

"Identifiable Medical Practices" (IMPs): Kovner, 45

Immigration Act, amendment: foreign physicians, 131
Immigration rules, labor department: foreign physicians, 131-132
Incentive and income, physician: fee-for-service practices, 70; retainer practices, 70; salary practices, 70
Incentive, leisure value: Pauly, 179
Incentive, marginal cost reduction: nonphysician, 58
Incentive physician: cost-sharing, 56-57; excess demand, 186
Incentives: alternative reimbursement schemes, 178; alternate reimbursement schemes, Sloan, 178; capital substitution, research needed, 190; capitation arrangements income, 60; cost and productivity, cost-sharing vs non-cost-sharing, 61; economic, manpower substitution, 30; equal income-sharing group, individual physician output, 59; fee-for-service reimbursement scheme, Monsma, 178; group practice managers, 181; institutional production, 67; physician productivity variations, Roemer, 185; physician services supply and demand, 185; practice modes, research needed, 192; revenue-cost-sharing, unequal shares, 60; salaried basis income, 60; salaried practice, 181; salaried reimbursement scheme, 155-156, 179; unequal income-sharing schemes, 181
Incentives and disincentives: prepayment retainer practices, Sloan, 181
Incentives, effect on: capitation practices, 62; equal income-sharing, 62; input purchase decisions, 54; lack of proficiency testing, 183; output, 54; physician performance, research needed, 192-193; practice efficiency, 54; price, 54; salaried practice, 62; unequal income-sharing, 62
Incentives, inherent effects: group practice, individual member, 53; practice mode, 54
Incentives, structure of: difficulties, cost and productivity, 66; group decision-making, research needed, 192; group practice size, research needed, 192; research needed, 76
Income: economies of scale, 173; gross, of dentists, dental output measurement, 109, 110; initial, partnerships-group, Jeffers, 81; initial, partnership-group, *Medical Economics*, 81; loss from price rise, 59; marginal income gain, cost-sharing, 56-57; median net, group vs solo practice, 47; net, income or profit equation, 55; salaried basis, incentives, 60
Income, physician, 46; capitation equations, 61; cost-sharing, 56; group practice output, 81; licensure, Sloan, 122; output, 81
Income and incentive, physician: fee-for-service practices, 70; retainer practices, 70; salary practices, 70
Income and licensure: medical schools, 122
Income and profit distribution: group practice, individual members, 63-64
Income considerations: group vs solo practice, 72, 77
Income-cost-sharing and cost-sharing: effects on group practice, 180
Income differences: partnership-group vs solo practice, 71, 73, 74-75
Income distribution: varying share of net income, Balfe and McNamara, 65
Income distribution methods: group practice, 65
Income equation (profit equation): total derivative, 56
Income equations: group practice, individual member, 58
Income incentives: capitation arrangements, 60
Income potential vs financial security, 72, 77
Income (revenue cost) sharing arrangements, 54, 55
Income (revenue-cost) sharing groups: group size and output, 62
Income-sharing: effects on cost and productivity, 57; effect on productivity, group practice physician, 49; effect on productivity, Sloan, 49; individual physician billings basis, 60; patient visits basis, 60; productivity, 49; equal basis, capitation equation, 61
Income-sharing schemes: Rorem, 65-66; unequal, incentives, 181; U.S. public health service, 65-66
Incomes (mean): by practice type, 71, 73, 74-75
Increase and decrease of productivity, 6
Increasing medical care costs: direct controls reimbursement approach, xiii
Individual vs group decision-making, 76
Innoculations, preventive care: Golladay, 168-169
Input: changes in productivity, 153
Input, market value as index: health care quality, 149-150
Input, physician vs aide, 7
Input, productive, managerial ability (technical efficiency), 11
Input, rates of: technical efficiency, 18
Input, "support": auxiliary personnel, 21
Input categories: health services, 144
Input coefficients combinations of, 5, 6
Input combinations: empirical vs hypothetical, 10
Input combinations and maximum output: production functions, 39-40
Input definitions and measurements: ambulatory care production, 13-14
Input-output: analysis of ancillary personnel, research needed, 189; health manpower substitution, Weiss, 154; indices, price weighted, 41; management, production processes, 32, notes; manpower substitution, 13; measured separately, 42; technical processes in, manpower substitution, 15; values, productivity measurement, 42; variables, in health services, 145-146; weighted sum-physician productivity, 40
Input-output coefficients: efficiency estimate, 9; estimation of, 9; identification of range, 9
Input-output equations: coefficient, 5, 6
Input-output measurement: health manpower, 145-146

Input-output relationship: health manpower productivity, 143
Input prices and rate of technical substitution: input utilization, 32, notes
Input purchase decisions: incentives, effect on, 54
Input quality: productivity, 195, notes
Input substitution: capital equipment, 155; economic feasibility, 155; patient self-care, 155; productivity growth, 155; rate of, 8; technical feasibility, 155; technical substitution, 32, notes
Input substitution, questions: ancillary personnel, 157
Input utilization: input prices and rate of technical substitution, 32, notes; rates of, production function, 8-9
Inputs: dental services, 108; health services, production function, 144-145; in continuous production functions, 16; physician productivity, 40; physician substitutes, 123; production function, capital substitution, 165; productive, marginal productivity estimation, 11; technical substitution, 29; value of, comprehensive prepaid medical group, 42
Inputs and maximum output: solo and group practices, 39
Inputs index, manpower: production function, 171
"Institutional licensure": allied health personnel, 132; health care institutions, 132; Hershey proposal, 132; individual physicians, 132
Institutional production incentive, 67
Institutions, health care: "institutional licensure", 132
Instruction, health care: see health care instruction
Insurance: Comprehensive Health, Health Maintenance Organization (HMO): effect on price index, health services productivity, 147
Intriligator and Kehrer: ancillaries and malpractice insurance premiums, 161

James and Wheeler: parent-care, 170
Jeffers: partnerships-group initial incomes, 81
Jewish medical students, proportion of: Bloomgarden, 125
Jewish physicians: discrimination, Kessel, 124-125, 126
Jews admitted to medical schools: Goldberg, 124-125, 126
Johannsen: patient noncompliance, analysis, 88
Johnson and Bernstein: dental assistants, limits and training of, 113-114
Jurisdictional disputes: physicians, 129
Jurisdictional restrictionism: DHEW licensure report, 128

Kaiser Foundation Clinics, Kovner: production function studies, 45
Kaiser-Permanente system: health care, and economic efficiency of, 86
Kegeles et al.: health care utilization in cancer detection, 90

Kehrer and Zaretsky: production function techniques, ancillary substitution, 157
Kessel: Jewish physicians, discrimination, 124-125, 126; licensure defined by output, 133; medical education reform, 133; periodic relicensure, 133
Kimbell and Lorant: economies of scale, Cobb-Douglas form, 172; production function techniques, ancillary substitution, 157
Kirscht et al.: patient knowledge of health care, 90
Klarman: definition of fractionation, 195, notes; *The Economics of Health*, health economic research, 152
Kovner: clinics studies, 32-33, notes; economies of scale, 48; economies of scale in productivity, 45-46; "Identifiable Medical Practices" (IMPs), 45; mathematical form of production function, 16; outpatient medical services, 45; outpatient production function, 48; production function estimates studies, 16; production function studies, Kaiser Foundation Clinics, 45; productivity and group practice size, 172

Labor department, immigration rules: foreign physicians, 131-132
Labor market: for allied health personnel, research needed, 189
Least squares bias: in estimated production function, physician hiring behavior, 18
Least-squares regression bias: empirical production function, 10-11
Leatherman: New Zealand-type nurses in developing countries and Australia, 112
Leisure, value of: effect of "group size" on, 66
Leisure value incentive: Pauly, 179
Licensed allied health occupations, 123
Licensed occupations: characteristics of, 120
Licensed Practical Nurses (LPNs): task delegation, 23
Licensing: equivalency qualifications, Dean, 183; maintenance of competency needed, Dean, 183; new health manpower categories, Dean, 182; 1910 Flexner report, 124; nursing mobility, 128; reforms needed, 128
Licensing, dental: state dental examining (licensing) boards, 113
Licensing, paramedical personnel: AMA and AHA, 128; Forgotson and Cook, 128; Hershey, 128
Licensing boards, state dental: dental auxiliaries defined by, 113
Licensing mechanism: American-trained physicians, 122; health manpower, 122
Licensure: acquired regulation theory, 120; alternatives, 121; certification alternative, 121; certification system alternative, Friedman, 132; consumer values and nonlicensed personnel, 121-122; controversy over, 119-120; cross sectional analysis, 134; defined by output, Kessel, 133; definition of, Dean, 182; DHEW: jurisdictional restrictionism report, 128; education and training requirements,

Licensure (cont.)
182-183; empirical verification of research needed, 193; endorsement, 136; foreign medical graduates, ECFMG exam, 130-131; geographical restrictions, 129-130; H.E.W. report, 126-127; health occupation competition, 128; health services productivity, 119; in general, Gellhorn, 135, notes; in general, Stigler, 135, notes; increase of chiropractors, 123; interstate variations effects on productivity, 184; interstate variations in ancillary utilization, research needed, 193; medical care quality, 121-122; motivation for, 121; of medical personnel, permissive, 121; original purposes and effects, 120; origins of, 119; physician, xv; physician supply, 120; price discrimination, competition, 135, notes; professional monopoly model, 119-120; proficiency and equivalency procedures needed, 183; public interest model, 119-120; regulations and medical markets, 135; Rottenberg, 120; simulation analysis of, empirically based, 134; simulation methods, noneconometric information, 135; time series analysis, 134
Licensure and income: medical schools, 122
Licensure and physician incomes: Sloan, 122
Licensure barriers: foreign medical graduates, 184; health manpower utilization, 184
Licensure condition variation and manpower utilization: research needed, 193
Licensure effects: costs, 182; manpower productivity, 181-184; physician and dentist mobility, 182; productivity, Frech, 182
Licensure law restrictions: ancillary personnel, 183; manpower substitution, 183
Licensure mechanism, control of: Pennell and Stewart, 126-127
Licensure, occupational: health care, 119; health manpower, 119; research needed, 133-134
Licensure reform: DHEW experiments, 133; policy issues, 132-133; productivity and costs, 133
Licensure restrictions: dental hygienists, 130; foreign-trained health workers, 130; health profession supply, 122; low-skilled wage levels, 123; Pennell and Stewart, 130
Licensure studies, origin of: Moore, 119; Stigler, 119
Limits to manpower substitution, 18
Lotzkar et al.: dental assistants study, 110
Louisville, Ky. Division of Mental Health study: dental assistants, 110
Ludwig, dental "technicians": efficiency, 111; quality of work, 111; training, 111

Malpractice: President's Commission on, ancillaries, 161
Malpractice insurance premiums and ancillaries: Intriligator and Kehrer, 161
Management: multispecialty groups, 63; production processes, input-output, 32, notes
Management, group practice, 54; compensation of, 63-64; cost-sharing, 63; decision-making surveys, 63
Managerial ability as productive input, 11
Managers, group practice: incentives, 181; reimbursement scheme preference, 181
Manpower, health: flexibility of medical care services, 29; full utilization of, 29
Manpower changes, medical: research needed, 193-194
Manpower inputs index: production function, 171
Manpower performance: value of training, research needed, 193
Manpower productivity, xiii, xiv; dentistry, 107; increasing, technical change, 187-188; licensure effects, 181-184; output weights, research needed, 148; output weights, strengthening market mechanisms, 148
Manpower quality changes: closer monitoring of practicing physicians, 156; educational structure, 156; selection of health professionals, 156
Manpower substitution: aides for physician, 21-22; ambulatory care, 3; data for output index, 13; delivery system, 29-30; description of task delegation, 15; deterrents to task delegation, 32; economic incentives, 30; estimates of continuous production functions, 15; licensure law restrictions, 183; limits to, 18; nonphysician medical personnel, xiv; outpatient facilities, 12; physician shortages, xiv; physician substitutes, 3-4; relative contribution of aides, 18; staffing patterns, alternative combinations, 20; "technical processes" in input-output, 15; three approaches to, 15; to increase productivity, 18; variation among medical inputs, 13
Manpower utilization: licensure condition variation, research needed, 193
Marginal cost, 55; imputed physician cost, 80, note; marginal revenue, 80, note; reduction incentive, nonphysician, 58
Marginal income gain: cost-sharing, 56-57
Marginal productivity: estimation of productive inputs, 11
Marginal products: production function, 10
Marginal revenue: marginal cost, 80, note
Market mechanisms, strengthening: manpower productivity output weights, 148
Mathematical form of production function: definition and equation, 17
Mathis: physician reallocation studies, 186
Maurizi: dentist productivity and technical change over time, 115, notes
Maurizi: production function estimates studies, 16
Measurement of improved health status: productivity, 42
Mechanic: patient sick role, 88; "sick role" and seeking medical care, 169
Medex: Physician's Assistant, 24
Medical assistants: as productive factors, 14; education and use, 14-15; task delegation, 23
Medical care: flexibility of services, 29; increasing costs, xiii, xiv; patient involvement, Golladay, 168

Medical care quality: licensure, 121-122
"Medical care vector": Reder, 42
Medical competition: prevention of Friedman, 126-127; Kessel, 126-127; Rayack, 126-127
"Medical conditions managed" Production function, 13
Medical Economics: description of task delegation studies, 15; group vs solo practice, patient visits survey, 48; partnership-group, initial incomes, 81; solo vs group practices, weeks worked, 71, 72
Medical Economics Incorporated survey, 44
Medical education: reform, Kessel, 133; research needed, 194
Medical group: productivity measurement, 42
Medical knowledge: development and transmission, research needed, 194
Medical output: definition of, 11-12; factors in measurement, 12; factors of medical services, 12
Medical personnel: permissive licensure of, 121; shortage, 53; three phases of activities, 45
Medical services: as output factors, 12; federal role, 53
Medical services produced: Relative Value Scale (RVS), 45
Medical schools: black, 124-125; discrimination, 123-126; expansion, 3; Jews admitted to, Goldberg, 124-125, 126; licensure and income, 122; raising physician quality, 187; students and graduates, 124-125
Medical students: proportion Jewish, Bloomgarden, 125
Medical treatment: patient noncompliance, 87
Minimum total cost function: production function, 41
Miyaska: health care utilization in cancer detection, 90
Mobility: foreign-trained health workers, Derbyshire, 130
Monetary variables and factor prices: returns to scale, 41
Monsma: incentives, fee-for-service reimbursement scheme, 178
Moore: origin of licensure studies, 119
Multiphasic screening, computerization: Garfield, 168
Multiple regression: parameters of production function, 10
Multispecialty groups, management of, 63
Multispecialty group practice physicians, 44
Multispecialty group practices: research needed, 49-50

National Center for Health Services Research: manpower productivity, xiii
National Center for Health Services Research and Development manpower productivity, xiii
National Health Insurance: increased, doctor "shortage", 3; physician "surplus" projections, xiv; plan including dentistry, xv
National mean charges: AMA, 67
Net income or profit equation, 55
New Jersey Dept. of Health, heart patients: patient self-care, 89
New Zealand dental nurse program: Walsh, 112
New Zealand program: "expanded function auxiliaries" (EFAs), 110
New Zealand-type nurses: in developing countries and Australia, Leatherman, 112; public dental services, 112
Newhouse: average cost curve, 47; average cost function, economies of scale, 173-174; cost sharing and group practice, 53; economies of scale, in group vs solo practices, 45; economies of scale, incentives, 173; output measurement, 46; production function variables, 46; variation in costs per patient visit, 67; X-inefficiencies, 174; X-inefficiency hypothesis, 46, 47
Noncompliance, patient: see patient noncompliance
Non-cost-sharing vs cost-sharing: cost and productivity incentives, 61
Noneconometric information: simulation methods and licensure, 135
Nonfee-for-service practices, 60
Non-licensed medical care: Stevens and Vermeulen, 122
Non-licensed medical personnel: cost of, physicians, 123
Non-licensed personnel: consumer values, licensure, 121-122
Nonphysician medical personnel: health manpower substitution, xiv
Nurse Midwife: improved use of, 23; Physician's Assistant, 24
Nursing: in individual health care instruction, Aiken, 92; in individual health care instruction, Cross and Parsons, 92; informal and individual patient education, 170; mobility and licensing, 128

Occupational licensure: research needed, 133-134
Office visits: group vs solo practice, 46
Operative dentistry: "technotherapists", 111
Optimum level of aide input, 18
Organizational changes: group practice, productivity gains from, 155-156; reimbursement schemes, productivity gains from, 155-156
Outpatient categories: output, 45
Outpatient clinics vs private practice: variation in costs per patient visit, 67
Outpatient facilities: manpower substitution in, 12; specialties in, 12
Outpatient medical services: Kovner, 45
Outpatient production function: Kovner, 48
Outpatient provider facilities: production functions, 12
Outpatient services: categories of, 45
Output, ambulatory care: classification of provider facilities, 12; definition of, 12
Output: auxiliary health manpower in definition, 14; auxiliary personnel in definition, 14; capital substitution, research needed, 190; definition of, ambulatory care, 11-12; economies of scale, 47; fee-for-service vs salaried practice, 71, 72; group practice physician

Output (cont.)
income, 81; group practice production function, returns to scale, 40; group practice size, 70; ideal vs actual rate of, 10; incentives effect on, 54; increased using aides, 23; input measured separately, 42; issues in defining, health production, 146-147; licensure defined by, Kessel, 133; market value of as index, health care quality, 149-150; maximum rates attainable, 10; measured as dollar value, 43; medical definition, 11-12; medical factors in measurement, 12; medical, factors of medical services, 12; outpatient categories, 45; patient visits, 47; physician income, 81; physician productivity equation, 40; solo vs group practice, 70; value of productivity, 150

Output, dental: see dental output

Output, individual physician: capitation equations, 61; equal income-sharing, group incentives, 59

Output, maximum: input combinations, production functions, 39-40; inputs, solo and group practices, 39

Output, rate of: see rate of output

Output, "real": demand conditions, 186; hospital use, Rafferty, 185-186

Output and group size: income (revenue-cost) sharing groups, 62

Output index: annual gross billings, 16; "conditions managed", 13; patient visit, 13; patient visit rates, 16; services produced, 16

Output maximization: constant returns to scale, 41

Output measurement: case-mix, 50, notes; case-mix, Rafferty, 50, notes; economies of scale, 46; Newhouse, 46; research needed, 49

Output measures: Reinhardt, 44

Output quality: productivity, 195, notes

Output weights: California Relative Value Scale (CRVS), 148; manpower productivity, research needed, 148; manpower productivity, strengthening market mechanisms, 148; relative value scales, Hughes, 148

Owens: solo vs group practice: weeks worked, 71, 72

Pamphlets: patient education, 91

Paramedic protocols: Reiffen and Komaroff, 167

Paramedical personnel: AMA, 123; physician productivity, 46; Rayack, 123

Parmedical personnel, licensing: AMA and AHA, 128; Forgotson and Cook, 128; Hershey, 128

Parameters of production function: empirical, 10

Parent-care: of patient, James Wheeler, 170; University of Kentucky Medical Center, 89-90

Partnership-group: initial incomes, Jeffers, 81; initial incomes, Medical Economics, 81; vs solo, income differences, 71, 73, 74-75

Patient: variables in willingness to utilize health care, 89

Patient care: visits per physician hour, 68-69

Patient compliance: Davis, 87-88; elderly, Curtis, 169; elderly, Schwartz, 169; research needed, 94; Simonds, 169

Patient contact time: pediatricians, 25

Patient education: see also health care instruction cost effective, research needed, 95, 191; cost reductions, 93; costs of, 93; economic implications of, 93; formal, Golladay, 170; group teaching, 91-92; Health Education Monograph, 91; informal and individual, advantages, 170; informal and individual, Golladay, 170; informal and individual, nursing, 170; methods, 93-94; motivation, 93; pamphlets, 91; strategies for, 91

Patient ignorance, effect of: health services productivity, 147

Patient instruction: formal methods, Young, 91; individual, Hallburg, 91

Patient involvement, medical care: Golladay, 168

Patient knowledge of health care, 90; Feldman, 90; Kirscht et al., 90

Patient knowledge: self-care, Golladay, 170; tuberculosis, Reinstein, 90; tuberculosis, Southworth, 90

Patient learning variations: Slowie, 91

Patient noncompliance: analysis, Johannsen, 88; causes, Preston and Miller, 87; causes and solutions, 87-88; chemotherapy, 87; Curtis, 87; factors, research needed, 95; factors in, 93; medical treatment, 87; physicians' perceptions of, Berkowitz, 88; reasons for, research needed, 191; research needed, 92-93; Schwartz et al., 87; summary, Simonds, 88; tubercular, Pragoff, 87

Patient participation: costs, 93; definition of, 86; economic analysis of, research needed, 94; education, xv; medical care system productivity, 85

Patient participation, cost-effective, 168; chronic problems, 93, 94; health maintenance, 94; research needed, 191; short-term episodic problems, 93

Patient participation in health care: behavior change, research needed, 190-192; economic implications, 94; research needed, 94

Patient role: health care, 92; self-care, research needed, 95, 191-192; utilization of health care system, 88

Patient seeking intervention: utilization of health care system, 88

Patient self-care: cost-effective programs, 89; diabetes, Charles F. Miller Hospital program, 89; diabetes, Ulrich and Kelley, 170; heart disease education, Rosenberg, 170; heart patients, 89; input substitution, 155; kidney, Peter Bent Brigham Hospital program, 89; mothers (parents) of hospitalized children, 89; New Jersey Dept. of Health, heart patients, 89; opportunities, 169-170; programs, 89; research needed, 94; Rosenberg, heart patient, 89

Patient sick role: Blackwell, 88; Mechanic, 88

Patient visit: management, staffing patterns, 20; overhead cost per, Taylor and Newhouse, 177; physician time studies, 33, notes; practice expenses (excluding physician) per, 177-178; rates as output index, 16

Patient visits: Allied Health workers and physicians, 26; delegated to PNPs, 28; group vs solo practice, AMA National Survey, 48; group vs solo practice, Donabedian, 48; group vs solo practice, *Medical Economics* survey, 48; measure of dental output, 109-110; output, 47; output index, 13

Patient visits basis: income sharing, 60

Patterns, feasible: task delegation, 33, notes

Patterson and Bergman: description of task delegation studies, 15

Patterson and Bergman: task delegation to AHWs, 23

Pauly: leisure value incentive, 179

Pediatric Nurse Practitioner (PNP): improved use of, 23; increased need of AHWs, 28; patient visits delegated, 28; physician telephone contact time; Hessel and Haggerty, 28; physician time saved, 28; replaced physician hours, 26-27; role of, 25; telephone contact time, 25

Pediatric office, Health Practitioner impact, 28

Pediatricians: patient contact time, 25; task delegation, 25; task delegation, ancillaries, 159; well child care, 25

Pennell and Stewart: control of licensure mechanism, 126-127; licensure restrictions, 130

Periodic examinations: economic efficiency, 87

Periodic relicensure: Kessel, 133

Peter Bent Brigham Hospital program: kidney patient self-care, 89

Peterson et al.: empirical studies of physician quality and performance, 187

Physician and dentist mobility: licensure effects, 182

Physician and PNP telephone contact time: Hessel and Haggerty, 28

Physician billings basis, individual: income sharing, 60

Physician characteristics, practice mode choices by: research needed, 192

Physician choice: geographical location, Yett and Sloan, 187; practice mode, 71, 73, 74-75

Physician demand, National Health Insurance increased, 3

Physician distribution: specialty-location, research needed, 193-194

Physician extenders: increased task delegation, 29; role of, 24

Physician hiring behavior: as least squares bias, estimated production function, 18

Physician hours, replaced: Pediatric Nurse Practitioners, 26-27

Physician incentive: cost-sharing, 56-57; excess demand, 186

Physician income, 46; capitation equations, 61; cost-sharing, 56; licensure, Sloan, 122; output, 81

Physician income and incentive: fee-for-service practices, 70; retainer practices, 70; salary practices, 70

Physician income and output: group practice, 81

Physician increased productivity: community size reallocation, 186; geographical reallocation, 186; specialty reallocation, 186

Physician input vs aide input, 7

Physician licensure, xv; method of, 122

Physician migratory behavior: Held, 187

Physician output, individual: capitation equations, 61; equal income-sharing, group incentives, 59

Physician performance: effects of incentives on, research needed, 192-193

Physician preference: practice mode, 72, 76; practice mode, *Hospital Physician* survey, 72, 76; practice mode, important factors, 72, 77

Physician productivity: average, Bailey, 46; factors in variation, 184-185; group practice, 53; incentives in variations, Roemer, 185; increase through manpower substitution, 18; inputs, 40; output equation, 40; paramedical personnel, 46; weighted sum, input-output, 40

Physician quality: medical schools, raised, 187

Physician quality and performance: empirical studies, Peterson et al., 187; research needed, 197

Physician reallocation: Crawford and McCormack studies, 186; economic cost, Sloan, 186; Mathis studies, 186

Physician reimbursement: productivity, 172

Physician service: excess demand, ancillary utilization, research needed, 189; supply and demand incentives, 185

Physician shortage: ancillary marginal productivity, 159; health manpower substitution, xiv

Physician substitutes: health manpower substitution, 3-4; inputs, 123

Physician supply: licensure, 120

Physician "surplus" projections: National Health Insurance, xiv

Physician time: per patient visit, 33, notes

Physician time saved: computer-assisted EKG, 167; computerization, 165-166; PNPs, 28

Physician use of time: productivity, Reinhardt, 153

Physician visits per hour: patient care, 68-69; productivity, 68-69

Physicians: aide utilization, 18-19; American-trained, licensing mechanism, 122; cost, non-licensed medical personnel, 123; demand curve, 55; discrimination of Jewish, Kessel, 124-125, 126; earnings, by practice type, 74; hospital, productivity, 175, 176; individual, "institutional licensure", 132; jurisdictional disputes, 129; limiting factor in production process, 18; nonutilization of auxiliary personnel: Human Resources Research Center, 160; opinions on task delegation increase, 160-161, 162-164; patient visits and AHWs, 26; perceptions of patient noncompliance, Berkowitz, 88; personal cost, cost equation,

Physicians (cont.)
58; proportion of women, Shryock, 124-125;
use of time in production, 19
Physicians, practicing, closer monitoring of:
manpower quality changes, 156
Physician's Assistant (PA): Child Health Associate, 24; Family Nurse Practitioner, 24;
health practitioners, 24; Medex, 24; Nurse
Midwife, 24; Pediatric Nurse Practitioner
(PNP), 24; productivity increase, Scheffler
and Stinson, 159; use of, activity analysis, 21
Policy issues: licensure reform, 132-133
Practice, by type: expenses per visit, 68-69
Practice efficiency: incentives effect on, 54
Practice expenses (excluding physician) per
patient visit, 177-178
Practice expenses per visit, 67
Practice mode: inherent incentives effects, 54;
physician choice of, 71, 73, 74-75
Practice mode, physician preference, 72, 76;
Hospital Physician survey, 72, 76; important
factors, 72, 77
Practice mode choices: by physician characteristics, research needed, 192; research needed,
77, 79; specific-deterrents, 76, 78
Practice modes: decision-making in various,
research needed, 77, 79; economic efficiency
of various, Frech and Ginsburg, 80, note;
incentives, research needed, 192
Practice setting, alternative: cost and productivity in, 66-67
Practice type: incomes (mean) by, 71, 73, 74-
75; physicians' earnings by, 74
Pragoff: patient noncompliance, tubercular, 87
Prepaid group practice plans, 196, notes
Prepaid medical group: value of individual care,
42
Prepayment effect: on productivity, 49
Prepayment retainer practices: group demand
schedule, 181; incentives and disincentives,
Sloan, 181
Preselected production function, 44
President's Commission on Malpractice: ancillaries, 161
Preston and Miller: patient noncompliance,
causes, 87
Prevention of medical competition: Friedman,
126-127; Kessel, 126-127; Rayack, 126-127
Preventive care: David, 87; Franco et al., 86-87;
Grinaldi, 87; innoculations, Golladay, 168-
169; major areas of, 168-169; motivation, 93;
Wade et al., 87
Preventive care costs: David, 168-169; Grinaldi,
168-169
Preventive health care: decrease in productivity,
151; presumed value, 92
Preventive health education, 87-89
Price: incentives effect on, 54; relative, 195,
notes
Price discrimination: competition, licensure,
135, notes
Price index: insurance effect on, health services
productivity, 147; productivity, 145
Price rise: income loss, 59
Price-setting in group practice, 58

Price-weighted input and output indices, 41
Prices: quality of health care, 150, 151
Primary care practices: allied health personnel,
159; task delegation, 158-159
Private practice vs outpatient clinics: variation
in costs per patient visit, 67
Private practitioners: production functions,
157-158
"Procedures completed per day": dental output
measurement, 110
Process innovation: production and technology,
156
Product innovation: Production and technology, 156
Production: analysis of, 4; dental services, 108;
group vs solo practice, Reinhardt, 172; physician use of time, 19; technology and process
innovation, 156; technology and product
innovation, 156
Production function, 7; average, 10; Bailey
productivity studies, 43-44; Cobb-Douglas
form, 172; Cobb-Douglas modified, 17; constant-elasticity-of-substitution (CES), 21-22;
constant returns to scale, 41; dental output,
115, notes; dual cost function, 41; economies
of scale, 171; effect of technical change on,
research needed, 194; empirical estimate, 16;
empirical, least-squares regression bias, 10-11;
equation defined, 8-9; health services productivity, 144; idealized, health services, 146;
importance of equation, 16; inputs, capital
substitution, 165; inputs, health services,
144-145; Kaiser Foundation Clinics studies,
Kovner, 45; manpower inputs index, 171;
marginal products, 10; mathematical form,
definition and equation, Reinhardt, 16-17;
maximum rates of output, 10; medical conditions managed, 13; minimum total cost function, 41; outpatient, Kovner, 48; parameters
of, 10; preselected, 44; processes in, 8; rates
of input utilization, 8-9; relatively most efficient, 32, notes; single, 48; solo practice, 39,
171; true, 44; variables, Newhouse, 46
Production function, continuous: algebraic
form discussed, 11; data collection and interpretation, 16; empirical estimates, 16-17;
estimation of various forms, 30; estimations
of, 10; inputs in, 16; research needed, 30;
unit of analysis, 16
Production function, estimated: physician
hiring behavior as least squares bias, 18
Production function, group practice, 171; economies of scale, 171; output, returns to scale,
40
Production function estimates: Boaz studies,
16; Kovner studies, 16; Maurizi studies, 16;
Reinhardt studies, 16
Production function or economies of scale: to
study group and solo practices, 41-42
Production function techniques, ancillary substitution: Bailey, 157; Kehrer and Zaretsky,
157; Kimbell and Lorant, 157; Reinhardt,
157; Reinhardt and Yett, 157
Production functions: ancillary personnel, re-

search needed, 189; input combinations and maximum output, 39-40; outpatient provider facilities, 12; private practitioners, 157-158; studied separately from production functions, 41-42; technical efficiency, 18

Production processes: combinations of, 8; economically efficient combinations, 32, notes; economically optimal characterization, 5, 6; input-output and management, 32, notes; physicians as limiting factor, 18; "n" inputs, 9; rate of output, 5, 6; Smith, Miller, and Golladay, 49; technically efficient set, 9; two input, 9

Productive factors: ambulatory care, 13-14; medical assistants, 14

Productivity: alternative reimbursement schemes, 178; average, 6; by group practice size, Bailey, 70; by group practice size, Yankauer et al., 70; changes in, input, 153; cost, Donabedian, 49; "cost and insurance approach", Reder, 42; definition of, 144; economies of scale, 45-46; economies of scale, conceptual difficulties, 172; economies of scale, Kovner, 45-46; economies of scale, Reinhardt, 45-46; effect of income sharing, group practice physician, 49; effect on income sharing, Sloan, 49; fee-for-service practices, 70; framework for definition, 39; group manager effect on, 49; group practice, 70; group practice, gains from organizational changes, 155-156; group vs solo, Reinhardt, 44; group vs solo practice, 48, 70, 170ff; health manpower, capital substitution, 165-168; health manpower, input-output relationship, 143; hospital physicians, 175, 176; identification of changes, 152-153; income sharing, 49; increase and decrease, 6; input quality, 195, notes; interstate licensure variations, 184; licensure effects, Frech, 182; measurement of improved health status, 42; medical care system, patient participation, 85; output quality, 195, notes; physician reimbursement, 172; physician use of time, Reinhardt, 153; predicted by simulation methods, 135; prepayment effect on, 49; price index, 145; production function studies, Bailey, 43-44; reimbursement schemes, gains from organizational changes, 155-156; retainer practices, 70; salaried hospital practice, 70; salary practices, 70; sources of growth, 153-154; total health manpower, 145; value of output, 150; visits per physician hour, 68-69

Productivity, ancillary marginal: physician shortage, 159

Productivity, decrease in: preventive health care, 151; technology, Thomas, 151

Productivity, dental: dental equipment effect on, 115, notes; increased by "expanded function auxiliaries" (EFAs), 110; nonlabor inputs and technical change, research needed, 114; technical change over time, Maurizi, 115, notes; use of dental auxiliaries, 109

Productivity, health services: insurance effect on price index, 147; licensure, 119; patient ignorance, effect of, 147

Productivity, increased ancillary substitution, 158-159, 160; Dental auxiliaries, 108; Dental technicians, 111-112; Physicians' Assistant, Scheffler and Stinson, 159

Productivity, increased physician: community size reallocation, 186; geographical reallocation, 186; specialty reallocation, 186

Productivity, manpower: dentistry, 95; licensure effects, 181-184; output weights, research needed, 148

Productivity, physician: see Physician productivity

Productivity, real-demand conditions, 186

Productivity and cost: "adverse selection problem", 66; alternative practice setting, 66-67; case-mix variation, 67; effects on income sharing, 57; incentive structure difficulties, 66; licensure reform, 133

Productivity and group practice size: ancillary personnel, 174, 176; Berki, 174, 176; effect on, 173; Kovner, 172; Yankauer et al., 174-175

Productivity decline: technical changes, 188

Productivity gains, 6; ancillary utilization, 160; use of ancillaries, Bailey, 164-165

Productivity growth: biomedical advances, Fuchs and Kramer, 153-154; health manpower substitution, 154-155; input substitution, 155; technological development, 154

Productivity implications: reimbursement schemes, Sloan, 180

Productivity measurement: input-output values, 42; medical group, 42; Reder, 42; service providers, 42

"Productivity spread": over specialties and geographic areas, 156

Proficiency and equivalency procedures needed: licensure, 183

Proficiency testing, lack of: effects on incentives, 183

Profit and income distribution: group practice, individual members, 63-64

Profit or net income equation, 55

Professional monopoly model: licensure, 119-120

Provider facilities: ambulatory care output, 12

Public interest model: licensure, 119-120

Quality: measurement of relative value scale, 151; new health manpower, research needed, 193-194

Quality, health care: market value as index, 149-150; market value of output as index, 149-150; prices, 150-151; value judgement, 149-151

Quality and limits: health care, 148-151

Quality and physician performance: research needed, 194

Quality index, health care: relative input prices, 150

Quality of health manpower: care and skill, 148-151; technical change, research needed, 194

Quality parameters: research needed, Reiffen and Komaroff, 189

Rafferty: case-mix as output measurement, 50, notes; demand pressures and case-mix, 159; hospitalization demand and cases treated, 185-186; "real" output and hospital use, 185-186
Rayack: paramedical personnel and the AMA, 123; specialists vs general practitioners, 129
Rate of input substitution, 8
Rate of output: ideal vs actual, 10; maximum attainable, 10; production process, 5, 6
Rate of input: technical efficiency, 18
Rates of input utilization: production function, 8-9
Research needed: ambulatory care production, 30; capital purchasing, demand pressures, 190; capital purchasing and reimbursement schemes, 190; continuous production functions, 30; cost-effective modes, patient participation, 191; cost-effective patient education, 95, 191; decision-making in various practice modes, 77, 79; dental output, 114; dental output mixes, dentists and auxiliaries, 114; dental productivity, nonlabor inputs and technical change, 114; development and transmission of medical knowledge, 194; economic analysis of health maintenance, 191; economic analysis of patient participation, 94; economic efficiency of health services, 143; education provided by group practice, 193; effects of incentives on physician performance, 192-193; effect of technical change on production function, 194; effects of technical change on quality of health manpower, 194; factors of patient noncompliance, 95; group practice managers, 192; health maintenance, 94; impact of medical education and training, 193-194; labor market for allied health personnel, 189; manpower performance and value of training, 193; manpower productivity output weights, 148; manpower utilization and licensure condition variation, 193; medical education, 194; medical manpower changes, 193-194; multispecialty group practices, 49-50; noncomputer based capital, potential, 190; occupational licensure, 133-134; output measurement, 49; patient compliance, 94; patient noncompliance, 92-93, 191; patient participation in health care, 94; patient participation in health care, behavior change, 190-192; patient role in self-care, 95, 191-192; patient self-care, 94; practice mode choice, 77, 79; practice mode choices by physician characteristics, 192; practice modes incentives, 192; privately vs publically developed capital, diffusion patterns, 190; quality and physician performance, 194; quality of new health manpower, 193-194; quality parameters, Reiffen and Komaroff, 189; specialty-location physician distribution, 193-194; task delegation, 30
Research needed, ancillary personnel: input-output analysis, 189; production functions, 189; task delegation, 189
Research needed, ancillary utilization: interstate licensure variations, 193; physician services excess demand, 189
Research needed, capital substitution, 168; economic feasibility, 189; incentives for, 190; output, 190
Research needed, structure of incentives, 76; group decision-making, 192; group practice size, 192
Research studies, synthesis of: delegation of tasks, 23
Reder: "Cost and Insurance" approach to productivity, 42; "medical care vector", 42; productivity measurement, 42
Reforms needed: licensing, 128
Registered nurses: education and use, 14-15; task delegation, 23
Regulations, licensure: medical markets, 135
Reiffer and Komaroff: chronic disease protocol, 167; paramedic protocols, 167; quality parameters, research needed, 189
Reimbursement schemes: capital purchasing, research needed, 190; capitation, 179; fee-for-service, 178; fee-for-service incentives, Monsma, 178; group practice managers preferences, 181; productivity gains from organizational changes, 155-156; productivity implications, Sloan, 180; salaried, incentives, 155-156, 179
Reimbursement schemes, alternative: incentives, 178; incentives, Sloan, 178; productivity, 178
Reinhardt: ancillary substitution, 154; economies of scale in productivity, 45-46; group vs solo practice productivity, 44; increased output using aides, 23; output measures, 44; physician use of time, productivity, 153; production function and specifications, 17; production function estimates studies, 16; production functions techniques, ancillary substitution, 157; production of group vs solo practice, 172
Reinhardt and Yett: production functions techniques, ancillary substitution, 157
Reinstein: patient knowledge of tuberculosis, 90
Relative contribution of aides: manpower substitution, 18
Relative input prices: quality index, health care, 150
Relative price, factors affecting, 195, notes
Relative Value Scale, California: surgery, Hughes et al., 174
Relative Value Scale (RVS): medical services produced, 45; quality measurement, 151
Relative value scales: as output weights, Hughes, 148
Renner: office visit health care instruction, 92
Research strategy: cost benefit analysis, Weisbrod, 194; disease treatment histories, 194; technological innovations, comparison studies, 194-195
Restrictions: foreign-trained medical personnel,

Stevens and Vermeulen, 131; hospital access, general practitioners, 129; hospital access, specialty boards, Stevens and Vermuelen, 129
Restrictions, licensure: dental hygienists, 130; foreign-trained health workers, 130; geographical, 129-130; Pennell and Stewart, 130
Resource-saving technology: disincentives, 188
Retainer practices: physician income and incentive, 70; productivity, 70
Returns to scale: monetary variables and factor prices, 41; output, group practice production function, 40
Returns to scale, constant: output maximization, 41
Revenue, marginal: marginal cost, 80, note
Revenue-cost sharing: effects, 53-54; equal shares, 57-59; unequal shares, 59; unequal shares, equation, 59; unequal shares, incentives, 60
Revenue-cost (income) sharing arrangements, 54, 55
Riddick et al.: excess demand, ancillary utilization, 186; utilization of auxiliaries, 159
Robbins: AMA educational standards, allied health personnel, 126-127
Roemer: physician productivity variations, incentives, 185
Rorem: group fee-setting practices, 80-81; income-sharing schemes, 65-66
Rosenberg: heart patient self-care, 89; heart patient self-care, disease education, 170
Rottenberg: licensure, 120

Salaried basis income: incentives, 60
Salaried hospital practice: productivity, 70
Salaried practice: advantages, 73, 77; advantages, Goldberg, 73; effects on incentive, 62; incentives, 181
Salaried practice vs fee-for-service, output, 71, 72
Salaried reimbursement scheme: incentives, 155-156, 179
Salary practices: physician income and incentive, 70; productivity, 70
Scheffler: group vs solo practice, 170
Scheffler and Stinson: Physician's Assistant, productivity increase, 159
Schwartz: elderly patient compliance, 169
Schwartz et al.: patient noncompliance, 87
Self-care, patient: see patient self-care
Self-care and patient knowledge: Golladay, 170
Service providers: productivity measurement, 42
Services produced: as output index, 16
Shephard: cost function, optimum practice size, 172
Shortage: dental manpower, foreign countries, 112; medical personnel, 53
Short-term episodic problems: cost-effective patient participation, 93
Shryock: women physicians, proportion of, 124-125
"Sick role" and seeking medical care: Blackwell, 169; Mechanic, 169

Simonds: patient compliance, 169; summary of patient noncompliance, 88
Simulation analysis of licensure, empirically based, 134
Simulation methods: productivity predicted by, 135
Simulation methods and licensure: noneconometric information, 135
Single: specialty group practice physicians, 44
Sloan: alternate reimbursement schemes incentives, 178; economic cost of physician reallocation, 186; group vs solo practice, 170; incentives and disincentives in prepayment retainer practices, 181; income-sharing effect on productivity, 49; licensure and physician incomes, 122; productivity implications, reimbursement schemes, 180; variation in costs per patient visit, 67
Slowie: patient learning variations, 91
Small practice, as opposed to clinic: flexibility of medical care services, 29
Smallpox innoculation education, 90
Smith, Miller, and Golladay: activity analysis approach to ambulatory-care, 20; production process, 49; task delegation to AHWs, 23; technological processes in medical care, 49
Solo and group practices: inputs and maximum output, 39; studied by economies of scale or production function, 41-42
Solo physicians: ancillary personnel, 157
Solo practice: economies of scale, 29; production function, 39, 171
Solo vs group practice: cost sharing arrangements, 46, 47; hours and weeks worked, 70-71; income considerations, 72, 77; median net incomes, 47; office visits, 46; output, 70; productivity, 70, 170ff; productivity, Reinhardt, 44; weeks worked, Medical Economics, 71, 72; weeks worked, Owens, 71, 72; work-weeks, 70-71
Solo vs partnership: group practice-income differences, 71, 73, 74-75
Soricelli: technotherapists, 111
Southworth: patient knowledge of tuberculosis, 90
Specialties in outpatient facilities, 12
Specialists vs general practitioners: Rayack, 129
Specialty boards: foreign citizens, 129; hospital access restrictions, Stevens and Vermuelen, 129
Specialty: location physician distribution-research needed, 193-194
Specialty reallocation: increased physician productivity, 186
Staffing patterns: alternative combinations, manpower substitution, 20; patient visit management, 20
State licensure examinations: foreign medical students, Derbyshire, 132
Stevens and Vermeulen: ECFMG exam, passing rates, 131; foreign medical students, law suit at Guadalajara U., 132; non-licensed medical care, 122; restrictions on foreign-trained medical personnel, 131; specialty boards, hospital access restrictions, 129

Stigler: licensure to general, 135, notes; origin of licensure studies, 119
Structure of incentives: research needed, 76
Substitution, health manpower: ambulatory care, 3; data for output index, 13; delivery system, 29-30; description of task delegation as approach to, 15; deterrents to task delegation, 32; economic incentives, 30; estimates of continuous production functions as approach to, 15; input-output, Weiss, 154; licensure law restrictions, 183; limits to, 18; nonphysician medical personnel, physician shortages, xiv; outpatient facilities, 12; physician aide, 21-22; physician substitutes, 3-4; productivity growth, 154-155; relative contribution of aides, 18; staffing patterns, alternative combinations, 20; "technical processes" in input-output, 15; three approaches to, 15; to increase productivity, 18; variation among medical inputs, 13
Supply, health profession: licensure restriction of, 122
Supply, physician: licensure, 120
Supply and demand: dental schools, 107-108; physician services, incentives, 185
Supply of dental care, 107
"Support" input: auxiliary personnel, 21

Task delegation: ancillary personnel, research needed, 189; deterrents to, manpower substitution, 32; feasible patterns, 33, notes; LPN's, 23; medical assistants, 23; pediatricians, 25; primary care practice, 158-159; registered nurses, 23; research needed, 30; synthesis of research studies, 23; time studies, 33, notes
Task delegation, ancillaries: pediatricians, 159
Task delegation, description of: approach to manpower substitution, 15; data collection and interpretation, 15; *Medical Economics* studies, 15; studies by Patterson and Bergman, 15; studies by Yankauer, Connelly, and Feldman, 15
Task delegation, increased: physician extenders, 29
Task delegation increase: physician opinions on, 160-161, 162-164
Task delegation to AHWs: Patterson and Bergman, 23; Smith, Miller, and Golladay, 23; Yankauer, Connelly, and Feldman, 23
Tasks performed: dental therapists, 110
"Tax deductible professional expenses": Yett, 47
Taylor and Newhouse: overhead costs per patient visit, 177; variation in costs per patient visit, 67
Technical change: effect on production function, research needed, 194; effects on quality of health manpower, research needed, 194; increasing manpower productivity, 187-188; polio research, Weisbrod, 187
Technical change over time: dentist productivity, Maurizi, 115, notes
Technical changes: productivity decline, 188
Technical efficiency: as productive input, 11;

production functions, 18; rates of inputs, 18
Technical feasibility: input substitution, 155
"Technical processes": definition of, ambulatory care production, 20; in input-output, manpower substitution, 15
Technical substitution: economically efficient combination, 32, notes; input utilization, 32, notes; inputs, 29; rate of, and input prices, input utilization, 32, notes
Technological development: productivity growth, 154
Technological innovations, comparison studies: research strategy, 194-195
Technological processes in medical care: Smith, Miller, and Golladay, 49
Technology: curitive and preventive vs maintenance, Thomas, 188; resource-saving, disincentives, 188
Technology, production: process innovation, 156; product innovation, 156
Technology and decrease in productivity: Thomas, 151
Technology of dentistry, 108
"Technotherapists": see also dental technicians, operative dentistry, 111; Soricelli, 111
Telephone contact time: Pediatric Nurse Practitioners, 25; physicians and PNP, Hessel and Haggerty, 28
Thomas: curative and preventive vs maintenance technology, 188; technology and decrease in productivity, 151
Time and motion studies: ambulatory care production, 30
Time series analysis: licensure, 134
Time studies: task delegation, 33, notes
Training, individualized: dental "clinical technicians", 111
Training and education: licensure requirements, 182-183
Treatment-need classes: values of goods and services used, 42
True production function, 44

Ulrich and Kelley: patient self-care, diabetes, 170
Unequal income-sharing: effects on incentive, 62; schemes, incentives, 181
Unequal shares, revenue-cost sharing, 59; equation, 59; incentives, 60
Unit of analysis: continuous production functions, 16
University of Kentucky Medical Center: care-by-parent, 89-90
U.S. Public Health Service: income sharing schemes, 65-66
Utilization of health care system: patient role in, 88; patient seeking intervention, 88

Value, dollar: output measurement, 43
Value, presumed: health care, preventive, 92
Value judgements: health care quality, 149-151
Value of goods and services used: treatment-need classes, 42
Value of individual care: prepaid medical

group, 42

Value of leisure: effect of "group size" on, 66

Value of output: productivity, 150

Value of training and manpower performance, research needed, 193

Values, consumer: nonlicensed personnel, licensure, 121-122

Varying share compensation: group size, 64-65

Varying share of net income: income distribution, Balfe and McNamara, 65

Visits, patient: as output index, 13

Visits per physician hour: in patient care, 68-69; productivity, 68-69

Wade et al.: preventive care, 87; undetected disabling diseases, 168-169

Wage levels, low-skilled: licensure restrictions, 123

Walsh: New Zealand dental nurse program, 112

Waxman and Rockoff: automated medical history results, 167; communications technologies in health care, 165; computerization, chemistry laboratories, 166

Weeks worked: group vs solo practices, *Medical Economics*, 71, 72; group vs solo practices, Owens, 71, 72

Weisbrod: cost benefit analysis research strategy, 194; technical change, polio research, 187

Weiss: input-output, health manpower substitution, 154; low-skilled health personnel, 123

Well child care: pediatricians, 25

Women physicians: proportion of, Shryock, 124-125

Workweek: economies of scale, 173

Workweeks: solo vs group practice, 70-71

World Health Organization, advice: expanded use of dental auxiliaries, 112

X-efficiency, 79, note

x-inefficiencies: Newhouse, 174

x-inefficiency hypothesis: Newhouse, 46, 47

Yankauer, Connelly, and Feldman: task delegation studies, 15, 23; utilization of auxiliaries, 159

Yankauer et al.: excess demand, auxilliary utilization, 186; productivity by group practice size, 70, 174-175

Yett: economies of scale, 47; economies of scale, cost function estimation, 175-177; "tax deductible professional expenses", 47

Yett and Sloan: physician choice of geographical location, 187

Young: formal patient instruction methods, 91

Zeckhauser and Eliastam: activity analysis, Physician's Assistants use, 21

About the Contributors

John Rafferty is Chief of the Economic Analysis Branch, The National Center for Health Services Research, U.S. Department of Health, Education and Welfare. He received the B.S. from New York University, University Heights, in 1962, and the Ph.D. in Economics from New York University, Washington Square, in 1970. He has taught Economics at Ball State University and at the University of Missouri. He has published a number of papers, dealing particularly with hospital utilization.

Uwe Reinhardt is associate professor of Economics and Public Affairs, Princeton University. He received the B.A. degree in Commerce and Economics at the University of Saskatchewan in 1964, and subsequently attended Yale University where he received the M.A. in 1965, the M.P.H. in 1967, and the Ph.D. in 1970. Since 1955 he has held a variety of positions in German and Canadian industry, and has served as a consultant to the federal government and to a number of non-profit research organizations.

Kenneth Smith is associate professor of Economics and director of the Health Economics Research Center at the University of Wisconsin. He received the B.A. from the University of Washington in 1964, and the Ph.D. in Economics from Northwestern University in 1968. He has served as junior economist with the Council of Economic Advisors, as Visiting Research Fellow at the Center for Operations Research and Econometrics, Université Catholique de Louvain in Belgium, and has taught at the University of California at San Diego.

Richard Scheffler is assistant professor of Economics and research associate in the Health Services Research Center at the University of North Carolina at Chapel Hill. He received the B.S. at the University of Vermont in 1965, the M.A. at Brooklyn College in 1967, and the Ph.D. at New York University in January, 1971. He is presently adjunct assistant professor of Economics and Policy Sciences at Duke University, has lectured in Economics at New York University, Hofstra University, and Brooklyn College.

Frank Sloan is associate professor in the Departments of Economics and Community Health and Family Medicine at the University of Florida. He received the B.A. at Oberlin College in 1964, and the Ph.D. in Economics at Harvard University in 1969. He was a summer intern on the President's Council of Economic Advisors, a Woodrow Wilson National Fellow, and has served as senior research associate at the University of Southern California, research associate with The RAND Corporation, lecturer at the Department of Economics, University of California at Los Angeles, and serves as an economic consultant to a number of government and private organizations.

Fredrick Golladay is assistant professor of Economics and a member of the Senior Research Staff of the Institute for Research on Poverty, at the University of Wisconsin. He received the B.A. from the University of Puget Sound in 1964, the M.A. from Northwestern University in 1966, and the Ph.D. from Northwestern University in 1968. He has taught at the University of Wisconsin, and has been an economist with the International Bank for Reconstruction and Development.

Paul Feldstein is professor in the Program in Hospital Administration and in the Department of Economics at the University of Michigan. He received the B.A. from the College of the City of New York in 1955, and subsequently attended the University of Chicago where he received the M.B.A. in 1958 and the Ph.D. in 1961. He has been director of the Division of Research of the American Hospital Association, and has served as full time consultant to the World Health Organization and to the Social Security Administration. He presently holds a number of consulting and advisory positions.

Harry Frech is assistant professor of Economics at the University of California at Santa Barbara. He received the B.S. degree at the University of Missouri in 1968, and the M.A. at the University of California at Los Angeles in 1970. He has taught at Montgomery College, UCLA, and the University of Missouri, and has previously been an economist with the U.S. Department of Health, Education and Welfare.

Jack Hadley is an economist with the National Center for Health Services Research, U.S. Department of Health, Education and Welfare. He received the B.A. from Brandeis University in 1968, and the M. Phil. in Economics from Yale University in 1970. He is currently completing requirements for the Ph.D. in Economics from Yale University.